ONE HAND CLAPPING

ONE HAND CLAPPING

The Story
of a Remarkable Young Man

Judy Andreas

FCP

Full Court Press
Englewood Cliffs, New Jersey

First Edition

Copyright © 2021 by Derek Domenici

Published in the United States of America by Full Court Press, 601 Palisade Avenue, Englewood Cliffs, NJ 07632
fullcourtpress.com

ISBN 978-1-953728-00-5
Library of Congress Control No. 2021923271

Editing and book design by Barry Sheinkopf

*This book was begun in 2004
and completed in 2007*

THIS BOOK IS DEDICATED TO ITS AUTHOR

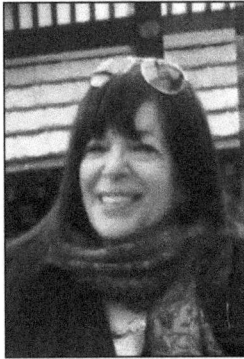

JUDITH B. ANDREAS
21 October, 1942–19 September, 2019

Though she is no longer with us to witness its publication, her fortitude and spiritual presence made it possible. After years of discussion, she transform events based on a true story into their fullest expression. I'm very fortunate to have been graced by her presence, and her voice will always be with me.

A resident of Suffern, New York, Judy worked as a social worker and a piano teacher. She loved her children, grandchildren, writing, volunteering, music, and people. She was fun and lively, had a great sense of humor, and will be very sorely missed.

—*Antony Risoli*

CHAPTER 1

THIS IS NOT MY STORY. *I am merely giving it a voice, a task for which I am grateful. The owner of the story is a remarkable young man named Anthony Risoli, my son Jason's friend.*

When I met Anthony, he was a mischievous youth with little direction but lots of charm. When I met him, he had two hands.

I will always remember the day of the accident. Jason and I were driving home on the State Thruway. Traffic was at a near standstill. As we rolled along, we wondered what had happened to cause the tie-up. There is no way we could ever have imagined that Anthony's motorcycle accident had caused it, or that his best friend would lose his right hand and forearm, and nearly his life.

There were plenty of fearful days at first. Anthony lay in a coma in Chimera Medical Center. Nobody knew if he was going to live. Through those uncertain days, Jason gave me reports about Anthony's progress. There were daily updates on how they were trying to save his limb, how he had to have screws placed into his head to alleviate the built-up brain pressure, when they removed skin from one leg to be grafted to the other, or how the ligaments from his thigh were also used to heal the motor movement in his arm; it seemed the list of procedures one after the other were endless.

I have read books about the power of prayer and believe that it is a key to the miraculous. At the very least, it lessens the feelings of helplessness and hopelessness.

Anthony's determination became an inspiration to me. As I watched his life take the shape of success, I knew that his story had to be told—because, contrary to initial appearances, Anthony's life was not ending, literally or figuratively. In fact, it was just beginning.

"What is the last thing you remember?" I asked.

Anthony looked off into space as if he were searching for an answer to my question. And then he began to tell his story. What follows are his words.

CHAPTER 2

OW MANY TIMES HAVE I BEEN ASKED that question? I've lost count. And though I try to answer it honestly, I can't be sure whether the memories are valid or part of the amorphous dream that followed my accident.

I had been doing wheelies on the State Thruway on my prized possession, my motorcycle. It was not the first time I had attempted such a daring feat, but I was an invincible twenty-year-old. Actions had no consequences in my universe. . .or so I thought.

What was the last thing I remembered? Perhaps the sound of brakes and screaming. Perhaps. Nothing is certain.

Were they *my* screams? I cannot be sure. I have fuzzy

recollections of being thrown into the air and then feeling a crushing weight before blackness began to envelop me.

I was airlifted to Chimera Medical Center, they later told me, where I spent the next two weeks in a coma. I was not expected to live.

What is a coma? I wonder.

Supposedly my body lay unconscious in a hospital bed. But where was my mind?

Sometimes a picture surfaces, and I wonder whether I have borrowed fragments and figments from friends and family, or actual memories are struggling to free themselves from the prison of my mind. Will I ever be certain? One thing is clear: That day in May changed the course of my life.

Anthony's eyes were looking past me. It was as if he were watching a drama, his drama, on a screen of his own making. I did not want to interrupt him. He continued:

I guess that everything was a blur for a long time. I can't remember a thing, not even a dream.

Where did I go?

And an even more mysterious question: How did I come back?

Then, one day, my eyelids began to move as if they were forcing themselves open. The light was harsh. I struggled to focus.

There was a silhouetted figure standing in front of a window with his back to me. As I blinked to clear my vision, I was able to recognize the outline of my father. What was he doing? Why was he standing there so still? Where *were* we?

"Are we in the Bahamas?" I asked.

My father turned to me. His usually stoic face looked drawn, sleepless. This man, who was the epitome of strength for me, appeared almost defeated. Was that a tear he was wiping from his eye? No, not my dad. He never cried.

I closed my eyes and recalled the day that he had first shared his stories with me.

"A man *has* to be strong," he'd advised me. "You know, son, I was only nine years old when I got that phone call telling me that my father had died. Did I cry? Of course not! I was a man even then. I had to be strong for my mother. My brother and I were now the men in the family, and we had to take care of my mom. We couldn't be walking around bawling like some little girls."

I opened my eyes wider. He was still standing there, eerily quiet.

I finally had to admit that something was wrong.

"Where *are* we, Dad?"

"We are in Chimera Medical Center, son. You had an

accident. You nearly died."

Chimera Medical Center?

This had to be a dream. "How long have I been here?"

"Two weeks."

"This is crazy. I feel fine," I said, trying to be a reflection of the man standing in front of me. I did not want him to know that fear had just entered the hospital room.

"Fine?" He sounded angry. "Didn't you hear me, kid? I said that you almost *died*."

I controlled my desire to argue. ."..What happened?"

"You were doing wheelies on the State Thruway at a hundred miles an hour. That's what happened."

"You've got to be kidding." My mind was so hazy. Sure, I had done wheelies before, but never on a heavily trafficked highway. I had always confined my antics to back roads and desolate areas.

As I fought to regain memories, a curious thought occurred to me. What if I *had* been riding on the back roads, as I usually did? What if I'd had an accident in a deserted area? How long might I have lain unconscious, waiting to be found? Perhaps this apparent act of idiocy had saved my life.

"You lead a charmed life," my father grumbled. "A doctor and a nurse were stuck in traffic heading in the opposite direction. They were on their way to the scene of a motorcycle accident on the opposite side of the Thruway. Their traffic had come to a standstill. It was then that they saw your accident and headed across the divider to help."

"What about the other accident?" I asked my Dad.

"Oh, that guy was already dead." My father did not look at me. His voice sounded shaky. "That could have been you, kid."

Is there such a thing as a coincidence? Before my accident, I might have thought so, but now I no longer do. Someone had lost his life that day in May, and my life had been spared. Why?

Dad's silhouette was still visible.

A strange question began gnawing at me. I had missed a final examination at school. Did that mean that all my hard work had been in vain?

." . .Dad, did I graduate?"

His expression softened, since my question seemed to have come out of nowhere. "Yes, you did. Your teacher told me that your grades had been so good that he passed you. . .even without the final examination. You graduated from Homestead Community College with a degree in business while you were lying in a hospital in a coma."

I began to laugh. Maybe it was merely a release of the tension I was feeling.

I looked at the man who stood at the foot of my bed, who had been both a hero and a villain in my life.

"How long have you been here, Dad?"

"The same as you have, two weeks. The past four days I slept in the hospital, waiting for you to wake up." His voice cracked. "They told me that you might not survive, but I knew you would. I knew you were strong. You are my son."

."..Where's Mom?"

"Tony, you know your mom. She's very fragile. She wanted to come, but seeing you this way would be too upsetting for her."

A nurse entered the room with alcohol, gauze pads, and a dressing. She began unwrapping the bandages on my leg. I looked down at the bloody site staring up at me. *Ughh*. I felt dizzy. It looked as if my thigh was missing.

"What's with my thigh?"

"While you were unconscious, the staff was grafting skin from your other leg onto your thigh," she explained.

"Am I going to be able to walk?" I could hardly ask the question.

"We think so." The nurse did not look me in the eye.

"*Think* so?" Was it a question or a statement? I was trying so hard to be strong, but inside, beneath that pretense, I was a frightened little boy.

Pictures of wheelchairs and crutches hung themselves on the walls of my mind. I blinked to clear the screen. I held back the tears.

"No," I said out loud. I was an active twenty-year-old before this happened, and I will be after. I am my father's son.

Later that night, the hospital room grew alive with visitors as friends and family began filing in to see me. I lay there laughing and joking with them as if nothing had happened. My fear was my secret.

It was on the following day that I started to feel pain. I yelled for the nurse.

"You've got to increase my medication. My leg is killing me."

In addition, the brace on my neck had been restricting my sleep, and I was cranky. "I need to *sleep!*" I yelled, trying to rip the damn thing from my neck.

They called me "insubordinate." "Anthony," said the nurse, "it will be far worse for you if you don't have the brace on. Trust me."

Her words annoyed me. Why should I trust her? I knew what was best for me. I always had. First of all, I had to get rid of the damned brace.

When the drugs began to wear off, I felt miserable. Everything hurt. I ripped off the collar, pulled out the catheter, and yanked the IVs from my chest. I had had enough of that place. I was getting out of there. I stood up, determined to walk.

The nurse found me lying on the floor. "What are you trying to *do?* You don't know how lucky you are to be *alive*. Do you want to kill yourself? . . . Don't you ever do that again, or I'll strap you to the bed."

Her words were harsh, but there was a twinkle in her eye. I knew I had frightened her. I also knew that she cared about me.

Much of the time I spent lying in that hospital bed, staring at the TV. If you had asked me what program I was watching, I probably couldn't have told you. I was too busy watching the drama inside my head.

On the third day, I noticed a change. It was as if the fog was beginning to lift and thoughts were getting clearer. In fact, it was the clearest I had felt since awakening from the coma. I looked at my left arm and saw that some skin was missing. Then I looked at my right arm, hiding under layers of bandages. Was it my imagination? It was shorter than my left! My heart started to pound. It couldn't be.

I compared the arms again. No. It was not my imagination. The limbs differed in length. But how. . . ?"

As I lay there studying my arms, my girlfriend, Jenn,

entered the room. She never made a quiet entrance. She bounded in with a big smile, holding a bag of chips while munching one loudly in her mouth.

"Would you stop that damn crunching?" I frowned.

"How are you feeling...or maybe I shouldn't ask. You don't sound so good."

"Did you know that I'm—I'm missing my hand?"

She continued munching on her chip. "Yup."

"*Yup?* What the hell are you saying? You've been visiting me all this time, and you didn't think it was important enough to mention that I had lost my right hand?"

"No. The doctors told me not to. They were afraid you might go into shock." Her voice quavered, and she stopped munching. Her smile turned downward. "Why are you *yelling* at me? It wasn't me who was doing freaking wheelies on the Thruway! But it *was* me who lay outside this damn place every night while you were in a coma. It was me who cried myself to sleep every night." Jenn's voice had gotten louder, and tears were streaming down her face.

Not knowing what to say, I meekly handed her a tissue. Visiting hours had ended, and the nurse escorted her out of the room. I shouldn't have yelled at her, but I was upset and I was afraid. She had merely been a target for my fear.

"Can I get you anything?" the nurse asked.

I wanted to respond, "Yes, another hand, please." Instead I said, "A pen and a piece of paper, please."

I wanted to see if I could write with my left hand. I also wanted to see if my brain had been affected.

She brought them to me. I don't know how long I lay there before I picked up the pen. So much depended on the results of the experiment I was about to perform.

Would the pen become an implement of liberation? I shook as I took it in my left hand. I steeled myself. Then I proceeded to write the alphabet. I could not believe what was happening. The letters were legible. It was *incredible.* My anxiety turned to joy.

I began to write phone numbers of people I knew. Yes, I could recall them. I wanted to leap from the bed and scream with delight! I was like a child on Christmas morning. Each thing I wrote was like opening another present.

Next I drew pictures. I felt high. With each pen stroke, the rest of my life started to take shape in front of me. My life was not over.

"Nurse, *nurse!*" I yelled. "I can *write.* I'm going to be OK!"

I continued writing until my hand grew tired. I even tried to draw pictures of myself. I must admit, they were not suitable for framing—but, to me, they were works of art.

CHAPTER 3

MY MIND WAS NO LONGER in the hospital bed. It was darting from past memories to future possibilities with little interest in the present. However, it was the "present" that was giving me the opportunity to better understand where I had been and where I was headed.

Perhaps someone else would have felt panic in my condition. Perhaps someone else would have sought counseling to help him through the pain of loss and the fear of the future. And yet, from as early as I could remember, I had never gotten any guidance and so, I'd learned never to expect any. I had learned to make my own choices, even if they had been poor ones.

Throughout my growing up, I'd marveled at how my

friends' parents would guide their children through the rough spots. My friend Kyle's parents were the best. Sometimes they would take me to the movies. Not only would they pay for me, but they would even buy me popcorn and a soda. What a contrast to my own parents, who were too busy stumbling over their own rough spots to even notice mine. My parents never noticed when their 11 year old son took a train into the City and went exploring. Would they have applauded me for figuring out the details on my own, or would they have punished me for such a potentially dangerous adventure?

Nobody cared if I spent weeks at a time sleeping at friends' homes. There was no concern as to where their son was or who he was with.

My school life was another area which passed beneath my parents' radar. "Don't ask; don't tell." They never asked and I never told.

The directional signals had been removed from their parenting vehicle and I had been handed the wheel.

Nobody went to "meet the teachers." Nobody looked at my grades. And though I lived with what appeared to be parents, I was virtually on my own.

When I was attending Middle School, my friends were all High School Students. During the school day, they were busily engaged in activities far from the "hallowed halls of learning."

My sixth grade teacher informed me that if I failed every class, I would still be moved to the seventh grade. What is that expression about "not looking a gift horse in the mouth?" There was no need to question. The proverbial carrot was being dangled in front of me and I followed it out of the school building.

The world was my education; the classroom was my jail cell. And so, during the school days, I joined my friends—roller blading, exploring the City and/or partying.

At the end of the sixth grade, I was bumped up to the seventh; F's or A's seemed irrelevant. The same thing happened as I left the seventh grade bound for the eighth; a string of F's dragging behind me.

I loved those days. The word "future" had no meaning for me. The "present" was my gift (present).

One day, however, my guidance counselor was able to get my attention. He issued a caveat "You'd better change your ways, young man. High School is different. You won't get away with this nonsense."

His words were momentarily troubling, but I quickly filed them in my mental refuse bin. "Who cares!"

When I entered High School, I had already been hanging out with senior class members and had a well earned reputation for being "rebellious." I deafened myself to punitive promises and admonishing actions.

I finished the 9th grade with my failure trail still behind me. "Art" was the only subject I passed. And so, I completed the 9th grade with one credit.

It was time to end this "High School Student" charade. I approached my parents.

"I want to drop out of High School."

They seemed mildly indifferent. I did not get any lectures or "stay in school" advice. And so, with my parents' consent, I said "goodbye" to my mandated curriculum at the age of sixteen.

You may find this difficult to believe, but I did have goals and dreams. I wanted to be salesman.

"Anthony, you could sell anybody anything." People noticed my gift, even in my earliest years as I stood in the hot sun selling lemonade outside my parents' home. Everyone who passed by wound up clutching a cup of Anthony's Answer to the Heat.

"Why would I need Earth Science or Math Courses to be a salesman?" I wondered. Yes, school was definitely irrelevant.

Freed from my High School prison, I enrolled in a GED program. The hours were perfect; in at 10:00 a.m., and out at 1:00 p.m. This left me free to get a job. Now

I could get on with MY life; a life of MY choosing. And, I would have money to spend. I was tired of always being broke. I was tired of begging my parents for some money and hearing, "Sorry, we don't have any extra cash."

CHAPTER 4

H OW MANY HOURS DID I LIE in that hospital bed lost in thought? That too will remain a mystery. And though I am not even certain what a "thought" is, I know that it was my past recollections and my future plans that kept me sane. It was my thoughts that energized me when I felt as if I were being tortured.

I would look back upon where I had been. I would wonder where I was headed. And I would plan and dream when feelings of despair tried to overtake me. My mind became my television as I watched the program of my life. Family and friends played significant roles in my drama.

I would simply close my eyes and watch different frames appear on the screen of my mind.

One recurrent scenario was played upon the backdrop

of fast food restaurants. I believe that I was around seven years old when I first became aware of it.

The family was packed into the car, heading through the MacDonald's Drive Thru.

"What is your order?" the woman said, looking confused.

"We just purchased an order, and you forgot to include two cheeseburgers, fries and a Coke," my mother responded.

The woman's expression changed from one of confusion to one of embarrassment. She was apologetic. "Oh, I'm so sorry," she stammered as she put the "missing" items in a bag.

Was it humiliation I was feeling? Something was terribly wrong. My mother was lying. And worse, she was stealing food.

I wanted to yell at my mother; to expose her. And yet, I sat there petrified. I was learning a lesson. One of my supposed role models was showing me how easy it was to lie and cheat. This lesson was one that would be repeated over and over again through my formative years by both my parents. After awhile, I began making excuses for their behavior.

"We didn't have much money. My parents sold hot dogs from one of those vending carts. They had to feed four growing boys. Who could blame them?"

The home in which we lived had beautiful woods across the street. I loved those woods and would escape there when things seemed out of control in my home.

The woods were not only a place for serious thought, they were also a place for serious play. My friends and I rode our four-wheelers in the woods, much to the chagrin of the local police.

One day, as we were riding along, we noticed a younger kid on his bicycle staring at us. My friend swerved causing the kid to run off the road. We kept on going without looking back.

"Oh-oh. We are out of gas," my friend remarked. "Let's go home."

As we left the woods, we noticed an ambulance and three cop cars speeding down the street. One of the cars began to chase us. We put our vehicle into full throttle, attempting the famous getaway scene. A second cop car blocked us off at the cross street. This officer meant business. He drew his gun and yelled at us to stop the engine. We were only eleven years old and, despite our tough exteriors, scared to death. He grabbed us and started yelling that we were going to jail because we had hit a child.

It turned out that the victim of our crime had been taken to the hospital after smashing his face on the curb.

This began a year of extensive reconstructive surgery for the poor youngster, and a year of probation for my friend and me. In addition, we earned an extremely bad reputation in our neighborhood. The "nice kids" were warned to avoid us.

I must admit that there were times when I deeply regretted what I had done. On those days, I would retreat to my sanctuary, the woods. I would battle with a barrage of sorrows that sought to surface.

One day, I noticed that they were knocking down trees across the street.

At first I felt sad and then I grew angry. A construction company was building homes. The land was strewn with lumber. I watched helplessly as they swallowed up my beautiful woods. What could I do?

DURING THOSE DAYS, MY FAVORITE PASTIME WAS roller blading with my friends. Dad had promised me that he'd build a ramp for us to skate on.

Late one night, he woke me up. "OK, son, let's go get some wood for your ramp."

In the darkness, we headed over to the construction site and loaded the trailer with lumber. That was the first of many midnight trips across the street where we helped ourselves to the lumber that the construction site had unwittingly provided.

When the ramp was finished, it was the hit of the neighborhood. All the kids were begging my dad to build them ramps. Despite the "borrowed" lumber, I felt really proud of my old man.

In addition to selling hotdogs, my parents also kept a supply of brownies on their truck. They told us kids that we could only eat the "kid brownies" but not the "adult brownies." I never questioned what the difference was.

One day, my grandmother came to visit. A plate of brownies was on the kitchen table.

"These look *good*."

"Those are adult brownies," I told her.

"Well, I'm an adult." She began munching away. As she ate, her behavior began to change. She started laughing hysterically and acting like a clown.

I had no idea what was happening. I was too young to understand that the "adult" brownies contained a secret ingredient: marijuana.

Later on, I learned that my parents had been selling pot alongside their hotdogs! I laughed out loud.

My mind was a morass of memories as I recalled coming of age in a world of deceit. My parents were my mentors and their teachings were not wasted on me. At a very young age, I too had learned how to scam the system.

And by the time I was seventeen, I was putting their teachings into practice.

It was the summer and I had secured a job in a large home improvement store. I'd been placed in the lawn and garden center and oversaw the sale of barbeques for their "summer blitz."

Selling, for me, was a piece of cake. A perspective customer would approach me to find out about purchasing one of the barbeques. I would rave about the features and fill his head with visions of burgers and beer. Sales were simple and straightforward.

To save space in my department, the supervisor had placed several assembled barbeques in front of the store. After the shopper had agreed to purchase one of the beauties, I would provide him with a product number. He would take the number to the cashier and pay for the barbeque. Then he would meet me outside, show me the receipt, and I would help him load his purchase into his vehicle.

At least, this was the way the scene was supposed to play out. However, the wheels in my brain were spinning as I imagined the wheels on a shiny new barbeque rolling into my parents' back yard.

I had a plan. My uncle was my test case. He entered my department, feigning interest in buying a barbeque. I smiled innocently and handed him a piece of paper. However, instead of writing the barbeque number on it, I left it blank. Next I handed my uncle a barbeque cover worth about fifty dollars.

He took the paper to the register and purchased the cover. Then he met me outside and handed me the receipt. I pretended to scrutinize the receipt carefully, just in case my supervisor was scrutinizing me.

Next, we loaded the barbeque onto his truck and he drove off.

It worked like a charm.

Word spread quickly, and before long, friends and family were coming to the store, buying fifty dollar barbeque covers and backing their trucks over to claim their five hundred dollar barbeques.

What a fantastic summer that was. Everyone I knew was enjoying burgers and corn on their beautiful new grills. The neighborhood was a veritable banquet. The air was good enough to eat.

THE HOSPITAL ADMINISTRATOR INTERRUPTED my thoughts. "I see you're in a good mood."

"I want to get out of here," I responded.

"You should be, in a few months."

"A few *months*? No way. Change that to one month.

A "few" months is too many. I want to start rehab."

I was raging. If I was going to walk again, I had to begin now. Each day seemed to be taking me further and further away from the life I had known.

CHAPTER 5

R EMEMBER THOSE DAYS WHEN The alarm clock would go off, and you had to roll yourself out of bed to get ready for school ? I hated those days and very often I'd hit the button and go back to sleep. However, the "wake up call" in the hospital dwarfed any screeching Baby Ben clock.

For here, in this hospital hell, I was awakened each day with a six-inch needle inserted into my abdomen. After that, the sponge baths, meals, medical exams and chaos of the day would follow.

One of the worst parts of my day, however, was not the monster needle. It was the sound of screaming patients and their crying loved ones. As long as I am alive, I will never forget those sounds. It was my own private house of horrors. I tried to keep to myself and tune out what was going on around me. It was futile, however.

"Hi," a voice called out, interrupting my silence.

OK, I thought, I'll stop being a recluse and behave.

"My name is Chip."

I wanted to reply, *What a silly name*; instead, I said, "Nice to meet you. I'm Anthony, Tony, or whatever you want to call me."

"What happened to you, Anthony?"

I began to explain my situation to Chip. Maybe it was good therapy to finally speak with another patient. And so, Chip and I started exchanging our personal war stories. Despite myself, I liked the guy. I began to open up.

"I had a stroke." His voice was slurred. "They put me in Intensive Care for a couple of weeks, but I'll be in rehab after this. I have two grandchildren, and I want to live to see them grow up. You're too young to know this, kid, but grandchildren are the best gift God can give you."

As his life unfolded, I learned that this was his second stroke.

"I've overcome this shit before, and I'll do it again." He smiled a crooked smile at me. "Don't worry, kid, life is full of miracles. You just have to believe."

Chip was soothing. I was grateful that I had been open

with him. I felt a lot softer and more optimistic as I put my head on the pillow to go to sleep that night.

It seemed as if I had just fallen asleep when I was awakened by the sound of buzzers. The room was filling up with staff.

"What the hell is going on?"

Curtains were slid open. An elderly man lay on the other side of me. I had grown used to his coughing but suddenly I was aware that he had grown quiet.

A voice began yelling, "We lost him! T.O.D."

"Chip!" I began to cry. "Someone just dropped dead!"

"At least it wasn't us, kid."

I couldn't take too much comfort from his words. I buried my head in my pillow so he would not hear me cry.

For days after that, I thought of the dead man. I wondered where he had gone. Did he have a family? Did he have Grandchildren? What were they going through? Was there life after death? I tried to voice my fears to Chip.

"Don't think so much. You'll find out the answers one day. Just be grateful that you are alive. I have learned to be grateful for every day. You never know when it will be your last. You never know."

Chip's words were not always easy for me to hear. My

mind would keep darting off in all sorts of directions. I thought about how young I was, how much life should be ahead of me. I thought about my goals and my dreams. Could he really understand that I was just a kid? I assumed that he was old. After all, he had grandchildren. Most of his life was probably behind him. And yet, with all my resistance, one thing was becoming clear to me: I looked forward to our conversations. What was it about this guy, I wondered.

Suddenly it hit me. *Chip was not afraid!* Could he be conning me? I didn't think so. No, he was the real deal. This man, with two strokes behind him had found peace. How had he done it? And why had life placed him next to me to help me through some of the darkest days of my life. Was this a gift from God? Was there a God?

"I know you are going through some really rough times, Anthony. I don't mean to make light of your situation."

"Thanks, Chip." I was glad that he could read my silence.

"What is your secret, Chip?"

"My secret? I have no secrets."

"I mean, why are you always so calm? The world is caving in around us, and you lie there at peace."

"Listen, Tony, when you've been through as many

things as I have, you realize that there are some things that are just beyond your control. Why knock yourself out? Life will present itself on its own terms.

"After my first stroke, I went through a lot of mental anguish, if you know what I mean. I was different then. I was worried. I had nightmares and would wake up screaming.

"One day, my youngest daughter visited me. She told me about a book she was reading in school. It was about an American Indian who was blind. Even though this woman had lost the ability to use her eyes, she could still see things. She called it 'inner vision.' She could even see into the future."

I was growing more and more confused. What was he talking about? I had heard stories of people who were psychic. Was that what he meant?

He looked over at me. "It's more than psychic." He seemed to read my mind. "This woman had visions. It's hard to describe. I'm not even sure that I understand. But there is one thing I will never forget. I even had my daughter copy it from the book."

He reached for a piece of paper that was on his night table.

"Listen to this, and don't forget it." He read, "Each day is new and we cannot keep the changes away forever.

We can only be thankful for each day we are alive. The tomorrows will take care of themselves."

I lay there silently, trying to grasp the meaning of what I had just heard.

"Chip," I finally said, "could you please give me a copy of what you read?"

"Sure, kid. Glad to help."

A long silence followed.

"Anthony, I may have some good news."

"Like?"

"The doctor ordered an EKG for me. I have a feeling that they're getting ready to release me."

Did you ever have one of those moments when you were torn in half? A part of me was genuinely happy for him. After all, getting out of the hospital was like graduating. Nobody wanted to stay confined in a bed a minute longer than necessary. And yet I was embarrassed to admit that I was going to miss him. Our conversations had helped me more than he knew.

"I am going to miss you, kid." He'd read my mind again.

"Same here." I swallowed my emotions, so that he would not see how deep they went. "Stay in touch, will you?"

"Sure. In fact, I want you to come over to my house

when you're walking again. I want you to come to a bar-beque."

A barbeque! I laughed out loud as I remembered the parade of barbeques exiting the Home Store that summer long ago.

"Did I say something funny?"

"You just brought back memories of a job I had. I would love to come to a barbeque at your home."

The pain in my arm was starting to grow intense. I yelled for the nurse.

"I need some meds! I don't enjoy pain!"

She entered the room with her favorite tool, a hypodermic needle. As she jammed it into my arm, I saw Chip being wheeled out.

"See you, Tony. See you soon."

Things were growing blurry. I looked up at the figures on the TV screen as I began to rise above my pain.

Ow! I thought. That woman on TV looks like my mom. . . . It *is* my mom! What's going on here? I saw myself standing near her bed. I couldn't have been more than eight years old. There was something really creepy going on. My mom's face looked all yellow.

"What happened to you, Mom?"

My father ushered me out of the room. "Watch what you say, son. Your mom doesn't want you to know she has been drinking alcohol. Pretend you don't know why she's sick."

I went back into the room and started playing a game I had grown very familiar with. I called it "Let's Pretend." Everyone knew what was going on. . .but everyone pretended they didn't. The game made me sick to my stomach but the rules were the rules. Anyone who broke them would be severely punished.

My mother smiled weakly at me. "I'm OK, Anthony. I just have some minor problems with my liver. I'll be out of here tomorrow."

Suddenly the scene switched to the kitchen in our home. There was Mom, sitting at the table, puffing on a cigarette. She smiled at me.

"How did you get out of the hospital?"

"It's easy, Anthony. You'll be getting out soon, too."

With a start, I opened my eyes. The room was eerily quiet. The television screen was dark. It'd all been a dream.

I glanced at Chip's bed to tell him about it, but he wasn't there. The bed looked freshly made, as if nobody had been sleeping in it.

"Nurse! Nurse! Where's Chip?"

"Who? How would I know? I just started this shift."

"He was the man in the next bed." I tried not to

sound panicky.

"Maybe the day nurse released him. You were sleeping for a long time, sonny boy." She shook her head. "They must have given you quite a dose of painkillers."

Sonny boy! Is that what she had called me? Nobody had ever used that term, and I didn't like it.

"Please call me Anthony," I answered curtly.

Suddenly the whole place felt cold and unfriendly. I remembered the nurse in *One Flew Over The Cuckoo's Nest*. Yes, Nurse Ratchet would be my nickname for this cold fish. Obviously she did not like me or maybe she just didn't like her job. Well, that was OK, because I didn't like her either.

I took a deep breath. What was going on? I did not even know this lady. Why was I so angry at her? And then it hit me. I was not really angry at her brusque mannerisms. The place had grown cold and unfriendly because Chip's warmth was missing.

Days would pass without a visitor. My friends had grown tired of battling the bridge traffic to visit me. The novelty had worn off.

I was bored and lonely and, with each passing day, I grew more and more irritable. Nagging became my new pastime.

"I hope I get out of here soon." I repeated that phrase

whenever I could grab the attention of a staff member. Maybe I could drive them all nuts. Then they would hurry up and transfer me out.

"Listen, Tony, you are going to be transferred to a rehabilitation center soon. We don't have a date yet, but just be patient." The male nurse looked tired. "These shifts are impossible."

"Lying in this bed is impossible. Wanna trade places?"

"It won't be that much longer," the nurse responded. "I understand that you'll be going to Fastline Rehab Hospital."

Fastline Rehab Hospital? Had he really said Fastline? I wanted to hug him.

"That's close to my home. My friends can start visiting me again."

CHAPTER 6

WITH EACH DAY I GREW MORE and more impatient. There was nothing fast about this Fastline business. What was taking so long? The dreary days dragged into weeks and I felt I was losing my mind.

Visiting hours were especially painful. I would lie there alone wondering if everyone had forgotten me.

"Hey, Tony," a voice exclaimed, crashing into my pity party.

"Billy! What the hell are you doing here?"

This had to be a nightmare. Billy was the last person I wanted to see. All of a sudden, my oppressive isolation seemed preferable to this snake that had just slithered into my room.

He kept a safe distance. "Sorry I didn't come sooner. I've been having all kinds of problems with my car."

There was a time when he and I had been really close and I would have done anything for him. However, a lot had gone down. As we grew older, Billy had become the consummate liar and master of the flimsy excuse. I was in no mood to listen to him. He might as well have been saying "blah blah blah." It all sounded the same to me.

"Did I come at a bad time?"

I felt like saying, "Every time is a bad time for you, liar." But instead I just muttered a soft "yes."

I lay there in silence while he stood uncomfortably near the curtain. Did he think I was going to strangle him with my good hand.

Suddenly, the curtain flew open, and a grinning nurse nearly knocked Billy over.

"Mr. Anthony! I've got good news. Your dream has come true. You will be out of here by the end of the week. You are going to the Fastline Rehab Trauma Center."

"Did you say trauma center? I thought I was supposed to go to the physical therapy amputee department."

"Sorry, Tony. The doctors just want to be on the safe side. They are afraid that the brain injury was much worse than the rest of the problems. They just want to run some tests."

Run tests? I couldn't believe what I was hearing. There was nothing the matter with my brain. I knew the alphabet. I knew my numbers. Why the hell did I need a trauma center?

"Cheer up. At least you're getting out of here."

"Hey, that's great, man," Billy interrupted "You'll be at the rehab center near Kyle's house."

"Billy, do you have a clue about anything? Do you know that Kyle came to see me? I heard that he even came while I was in my coma. He didn't let any—ahem—'car trouble' stop him, since he doesn't even have a car. So, let's stop the shit. Billy, I almost died. Or maybe you would have been happy if I did. Then you wouldn't have to pay me all the money you owe me. Or were you hoping that my accident had wiped out my memory?"

He stammered, "I'm going to pay you back, man."

"Visiting hours are over," the nurse made a perfect entrance.

"When am I going to get my money?" I wasn't going to let the snake wriggle out so easily.

"Tony, work with me. You'll get it. You know me."

Yes, I knew him, and that was the problem. Billy's name was prominently entered in the ledger of people who owed me money.

CHAPTER 7

MY WHEELCHAIR COULD HAVE BEEN a Jaguar as I sped through the doors of the Chimera Medical Center bound for Fastline. Only once did I turn around.

"Goodbye forever!" I waved at the building.

"Goodbye." A man stood near the front door waving back at me.

"Chip! Is that you?"

The man shook his head. "Sorry, son. You've got me confused with someone else."

I choked back the emotions I was feeling. Today was one day I did not want to feel depressed.

They placed me in an ambulance and we slowly drove to my new habitat, Fastline. Even though I was not happy with the idea of spending another month in a hospital, especially in a trauma center, I was thrilled that I would be only minutes away from my friends and family.

We pulled up to the rehab hospital and they wheeled me out. I noticed people walking into the place carrying balloons and flowers.

They must be bringing these gifts to their loved ones, I thought. At that moment I would have given anything for someone to present me with a token of their care and concern. I closed my eyes and pictured a huge bunch of balloons with the words *Welcome Back, Tony*. I pictured my family and friends smiling at me. Was I setting myself up for another disappointment? Was I just torturing myself?

The attendant wheeled me into the elevator. I watched the buttons light up as we passed the third floor amputee department and headed to the fifth floor trauma department.

They placed me in my hospital bed which was separated from other patients by curtains, much like the Chimera Center I had just left.

That night I could not sleep. I kept thinking of the people I most wanted to see.

My thoughts turned to Kyle. I thought about how his parents had given him everything he wanted. I thought about how ungrateful he had been. Even with such a wonderful, supportive family, Kyle had bummed around town focusing on drugs and alcohol. How many times had I wished Kyle would "see the light"? How many times had I wished that he would change his losing ways? How many times did I wish he would appreciate the wonderful family he had? But, the most important thing, for me, was that I knew Kyle cared about me. When things were really unbearable, Kyle was a true friend. I couldn't wait to see him.

"I've got to see Rob, too," I said out loud. There were so many questions I needed to ask him.

You see, he and three other friends had been with me on the State Thruway the day of the accident. Rob had witnessed the whole thing. And though I had heard third and fourth hand accounts of what happened, I had never gotten a chance to find out exactly what he saw. I desperately needed to speak to him.

I felt as if my brain hurt. My mind was racing and I needed to sleep. I wanted to get away from my thoughts. It was as if my head was going to burst.

"Nurse, can you give me something to help me sleep?"

She appeared with her magic pills, and I entered the welcome haze.

Then I heard a voice in my head and saw an image of

Rob pulling down his helmet screaming out loud as I performed a wheelie at 100 mph. "That was fucking awesome, man!"

He and my three other friends were applauding. I was their hero.

"Check this out." It was time to try something new. This would stun everyone. I pulled the front end of my motorcycle up at 70 mph and rode it out until I reached 120.

It was then that my audience witnessed the most theatrical motorcycle accident they had ever seen. As I hit the concrete of the State Thruway, I was thrown like a rag doll and skidded a tenth of a mile to my standstill. Suddenly the doctor and nurse appeared.

"I'll call for a helicopter." The doctor's voice was breathless.

Was I dreaming? I was so confused. It all seemed so real. What kind of meds had that nurse given me?

"Hey, bro, what's good?" Who was that voice? Was it part of the dream? I looked towards the door.

"Oh, shit! Rob! Where the hell have you been?"

"Anthony, I was at the hospital the day after the accident. After that it was almost impossible for me to get back to that place. Thanks for moving closer, bro."

"Rob, I've been going nuts. I don't even know where

to begin. I want to hear exactly what happened the day of the accident. I have been struggling with bits and pieces, and it's driving me insane."

My heart began pounding as he relayed the whole gruesome story of what had transpired.

Even though I had asked for every detail, by the time he finished, I was exhausted. I felt as if I had just relived the nightmare.

"Sorry, man, but you asked."

"Don't be sorry," I assured him. "I needed to hear what you had to say. And now I need to be alone for awhile."

It was time to put the accident to rest along with my tired body. Rob left just as visiting hours ended.

CHAPTER 8

T HE SUN SHONE BRIGHTLY THROUGH my hospital window, beckoning me to come outside. "Nurse! When am I going to start walking?"

"My, you *are* in a hurry, aren't you? Today is the day that you begin your rehabilitation. After a week of rehab, we will be in a better position to evaluate your progress. You are going to be meeting with the Neurologist today. His name is Dr. Smith and he's really tops in the field. You'll like him."

"Oh, sure." I'd let my sarcasm slip out.

The door opened, and in wheeled the usual hospital slop euphemistically called "lunch."

"What's for lunch?" I tried to act as if this gunk on the approaching tray was authentic food.

"It's baloney and cheese sandwiches, made to perfection"

I felt myself gagging.

Baloney! That was a word I had heard time and time again from my grandmother. I used to think it meant "nonsense" or "nothing important." However, "baloney" had another meaning in my youth.

I recalled the distinct odor that used to permeate my home.

"What's that smell?" I would innocently ask my mother the cook.

"Oh, it's just baloney."

One day, I was visiting a friend and there was that fetid odor again. "Are you making baloney?" I asked.

He laughed. "You've never smelled crack, Tony?"

With one sentence, both my friend and my parents had fallen from grace, although it was not a very long trip.

I never mentioned my revelation to my parents. It was time to continue our "Let's Pretend" game. In fact, I have never told anyone about this incident until now. I kept it in my mental file cabinet, buried in the deceit folder.

"Nurse! Can I get something else?"

"What's the matter, Tony? Don't you like our choice baloney cuts?"

"Actually, I cannot eat baloney. It makes me sick.

Please take it away."

"Well, I think we have some turkey sandwiches that aren't too old." She laughed. "I'll get you one."

She reappeared with what looked like filet mignon. Never had turkey seemed so appetizing. I wolfed it down as the attendant entered.

"Time for business?"

"What kind of business?" I asked.

"I was told that you have an appointment with the neurologist now. I'm going to wheel you there."

"Ah yes, the top-notch Dr. Smith. His reputation has preceded him."

The attendant frowned. "Actually, I was told to take you to see Dr. King."

"Dr. King? Is he royalty?"

"Huh?" The attendant was not enjoying my sense of humor. He quickly wheeled me down the corridor.

A LARGE MAN WAS SITTING IN A LARGE CHAIR, or was it a throne? "You must be Dr. King."

"Oh, no. Dr. King is tied up with other patients. I will be working with you instead." He leaned over his abundant belly and handed me some reading material. "Read this out loud, big guy."

"O.K," I responded, "but could you please do me a

favor and don't call me 'big guy'?" It was one of those pot calling the kettle black moments. "Also, before we begin, I have gotta ask you something? What kind of a doctor are you?"

"I'm a resident in the neurology department. I'm going to go through some standard questions with you."

"A resident? Isn't that like a student?"

"Look, buddy, you don't need to be Einstein to ask these questions. They are standard protocol. Any jackass can do this."

I stifled my wisecrack. Instead I asked, "Sir, when I finish with the 'standard protocol,' will I be able to begin my physical therapy?"

"After a few more meetings, I am sure you'll be ready. A lot depends on how well you do on these tests."

An hour went by, and I shot off the answers like a pro. I knew my name, what country I lived in, how old I was, and even what it felt like to ride a four-wheeler with two hands. I was amazing Dr. Resident with my genius, or so I thought.

And yet, each day, I was called back to the clinic, where a whole new round of questions was fired at me.

I couldn't help but wonder whatever had happened to Drs. Smith and King. Did these "top-notch" doctors only deal with people they deemed were "top-notch" patients?

But though I acted disgusted, I must admit that I had begun to look forward to my meetings with the large jolly man. It certainly was better than lying in bed or watching some daytime garbage on television. But mainly, after we finished playing "Evaluate Tony's Trauma," visiting hours began.

CHAPTER 9

VISITING HOURS HAD BECOME a daily party. More and more friends began dropping by. The word had gotten out and Fastline had morphed into a fast lane.

I especially loved when Darlene, came to visit. She and I had met on the bus when we were in elementary school. We liked one another immediately and began exchanging stories of our families. I felt that I had met my female counterpart. We had similar upbringings and had never learned to respect others or to play by the rules.

One night she entered my room with her face buried in a chicken parmesan hero sandwich. I began to drool.

"Darlene, you're killing me. Do you know how long it's been since I've had anything that resembled food?"

"Try some of this?" She waved the sandwich under my flaring nostrils.

"Hey! Keep that down! I think I am supposed to be on a special diet of Styrofoam. Lower that sandwich, and don't let the nurse see it. In fact, wrap in it this roll of gauze."

"Tony, that looks ridiculous. And what are you going to do about the smell?"

"I'll have it finished before the nurse comes in." I shoved a large piece down my throat and started choking.

She came in "Easy, Tony." The nurse was not on cue that night. "Are you OK? And what's that smell in here?"

I'd hidden the remains of the sandwich under the blanket.

"Are you hungry, Tony?" She was overplaying her role. "I can bring you some lemon Jell-O if you want."

Lemon Jell-O? I still had my teeth. "No, thanks. Though it does sound yummy, I'm full. By the way, did I happen to mention that the meatballs were excellent tonight? That was meat in those balls, wasn't it?"

"You are so funny." She headed towards the door. "Be good, kiddies."

"Kiddies? How can you stand it here, T.?"

"Forget this place, Darlene. You're supposed to be

here to take my mind off it."

Darlene was a year older than I was, but we shared that same string of F's in Middle School. We used to refer to one another as "failure" and "fuck-up." But most of all, we called each other "friend."

Perhaps it was that we were both from poor families, but it hadn't been long before we were fast friends.

Darlene, like me, had a good business sense at an early age.

"What can we do to make money?" Her brain never stopped.

We began with the basics: selling overpriced candy bars and cookies to our richer classmates. It was a business doomed to fail. After all, our potential customers hadn't fallen off the cabbage truck, nor did they fall for the inflated prices. We had to find a more desirable product.

Meanwhile, the school had placed our dear friend Kyle on Ritalin. They told his parents that he was out of control, and the little pill would help him focus. However, it was explained quite emphatically that the pill only worked for people who had Kyle's learning disability. If anyone else dared to use it, they might experience a "high" feeling, which could be quite frightening. In addition, the students were warned that snorting it through the nose would increase that frightening feeling of being "high."

"High," eh? The word "frightening" got lost in the sentence, and the admonition quickly became an invitation. It wasn't long before Kyle's friends were helping themselves to Kyle's little helpers.

Darlene and I had finally found our perfect product. Kyle was glad to get rid of the pills, and we were glad to take them off his hands. The wealthy kids were glad to pay us to get it down their throats. And so, for awhile, we made good money.

However, this business venture was also doomed to failure. It seems that attention deficit disorder, or whatever Kyle was suffering from, had become pandemic. The school was prescribing these little pills to everyone who squirmed. The supply had grown greater than the demand, and ,once more, Darlene and I sadly hung up our "out of business" sign. For a month or two, we were broke, disgusted and out of ideas.

As a last resort, I had finally taken a respectable job at a car wash. However, it did not do much for my ego cleaning the grime off friends' Beemers.

One day, Darlene knocked wildly on my door.

"What's up?"

Her face had been glowing. "Tony, we are back in business."

The words had poured from her mouth in a wave of enthusiasm.

She explained how her old friend Jerry was supporting himself in California. "He's growing mushrooms!" she squealed. "You know what I'm talking about? Magic mushrooms. He's making a great living, and he's agreed to send some back East."

Thanks to my earlier education in the DARE classes, I had been introduced to the supposed dangers of the "shrooms." But for me, real learning took place through first-hand experience. After a bit of experimentation, I became quite savvy about mushrooms and their effects on the mind. However, I wasn't certain whether this was a good *career* move.

It was time to survey my peers. After all, they were the prospective consumers, weren't they?

I 'dapproached Kyle. He was an easy sell.

So he and I had decided to go into the mushroom business. I'd told Darlene to contact Jerry, that we would begin our Magical Mystery Mushroom Market.

"Tony, are you going to eat that chicken parm?" Darlene asked, and I was back in the present.

"It's going to taste like hell."

"Just like the rest of the food around here."

"Sorry, Darlene, I was thinking of Jerry. Man, we had

some good times. What's Jerry up to?"

"Look, Tony." Darlene introduced a serious note into my psychedelic symphony. "Those days are gone."

I noticed that her voice had become barely audible as the nurse came bouncing into the room. Efficiently, she began fluffing my pillow and fussing with my blankets.

"Tony!" Where did this chicken hero sandwich come from? Or maybe that's a silly question, when you left a Denato's bag under your bed."

"Sorry, Nurse." Darlene came to the rescue. "I brought it to him. I didn't mean to break any dietary rules. "

"Naughty, naughty," the nurse scolded. "Our young friend is on a strict diet. Only healing foods are permitted."

"Ah, yes. The healing baloney slices nestled between two fluffy pieces of Wonder Bread."

"I had better get going, T." Darlene headed for the door. "See you."

That night was probably the first time since my accident that I felt the stresses of the outside world begin to creep into my hospital room. No longer was I focusing on my missing limb and my disabled leg. My thoughts were now speeding down a track towards a station marked "future." I thought about my finances, my belongings, my apartment—all the "stuff" that I had buried in the recesses of my mind. How was I going to replace what had taken me so long to accumulate? I had to get out of there. I couldn't sit like a zombie responding to daily dumb-ass questions any longer. I was fed up with hearing, "You're doing very well, Tony." If I was doing so well, then I needed to be released; not in a month or in a week. . .but *now*.

Sleep no longer offered me any relief. Dreams had been replaced by nightmares and I would awaken more exhausted than when I had lain down.

I fantasized about wiping the smiles off the nurses' faces, and I was fantasizing about answering Dr. "Big Boy's" questions with baby talk, if I did not fear that they would lock me up.

I would daydream about the city, where I had pursued my youthful explorations. I could even feel the pavement under my feet and hear the sounds of the proverbial hustle and bustle. I loved that place and planned to move there when my recovery was complete. Perhaps I would attend school there. Yes, I would get a degree in sales or marketing or whatever they offered. Who knew? Maybe I would become very rich and work on Wall Street.

One night I dozed off thinking about the winding streets and quaint little shops. Suddenly a homeless man fell out of a doorway onto my path. Fear gripped me. I walked faster, but now homeless people were surrounding me. I woke up screaming.

"Mr. Risoli? Is everything OK?" An unfamiliar face had joined the night shift.

"Yes. It was just a dream, nurse."

"Do you have these night terrors frequently?"

"Nope. . .first time. My usual dreams about candy canes and carousels were beginning to bore me."

Sometimes I wondered whether the hospital had added extra hours to the days. Was it possible that time could move so slowly? I could not believe that only three days had passed when Dr. Big Boy looked me in the eye and said those words I had been aching to hear. "Tony, I am going to sign you out. You have done swimmingly on your test responses."

"Swimmingly? Thanks, sir, I guess."

"Trauma treatment testing is terminated, Tony." (He certainly was a clown.)

The following day, an attendant came to transport me.

"Where are we going? I thought I had graduated from trauma testing."

The attendant looked at his clipboard. "Today you are going to see Dr. Smith. At least, that's what my instructions say." He double checked his memo. "Yup, Dr.

Smith it is."

"Why the change? Is he going to ask me a more challenging battery of questions?"

"I think you'll be really happy to meet Dr. Smith. You know, he's top-notch in the field."

"Well, tell him to come in from the field."

"What?"

"Oh, never mind."

DR. SMITH SHOOK MY HAND and showed me a piece of paper on which the words *Memory loss, not memory damage* were printed.

In layman's terms, I was told that my memory could be totally regained. I was well on the road to recovery and on the road out of the trauma center.

The attendant wheeled me into the elevator. I smiled happily as it stopped at the amputee floor.

I surveyed the surroundings. The walls were decorated with colorful posters depicting missing limbs. My chair was wheeled past a curtain through which half a leg was extended. I know you will find this hard to believe, but the potentially grotesque sight was strangely comforting. I was finally in the amputee department.

They lifted me into my new bed. It was similar to the ones that had preceded it, but that was only the appearance. I was finally making progress, and I knew that it wouldn't be long before I was sleeping in my own bed and the nightmares and daymares had ended.

"Someone will be with you shortly to take you to meet the occupational therapist. You will be learning scar management, desensitization, and having physical therapy to strengthen the muscle in your arm."

That "someone" turned out to be a woman named Marly. She was one of a bevy of beauties in the Occupational Therapy department. Maybe I had died and gone to heaven.

"You will be meeting with a prosthetist." Marly smiled.

"A prostitute?"

"Tony! Behave yourself. A prosthetist is a certified practitioner of prosthetics. He is going to evaluate you to see if you are a good candidate for a prosthesis."

I was beginning to wish I had access to Google. These terms were confusing, and I did not want to appear ignorant.

"I know it's a lot of new words, Tony, but you are beginning a whole new phase of your life,"

Meeting with Marly and her well-endowed staff made life in physical therapy quite enjoyable. When I wasn't munching on eye candy, I was working hard at the exercises. In a short time, my arm had grown noticeably stronger.

I was told that I was ready for outpatient therapy.

Marly entered my room.

"You are leaving tomorrow, Tony. Your parents will be picking you up in the morning."

"Are you coming with me?"

Marly continued talking as if she had not heard me. She had definitely learned to tune me out. "A nurse will be coming to your home three times a week. She'll be dressing your leg wounds and teaching you more arm strengthening exercises."

I was overcome with gratitude.

"Will the nurse be as pretty as you, Marly?"

"Tony, you are incorrigible. With all your wisecracking, I almost forgot what I wanted to tell you. Listen to this. I took a course that I thought would be perfect for you to attend. It was geared to teaching occupational therapists to work with patients prior to their receiving a myo-electric prosthesis."

"Speak English, Marly. What is a myo-electric prosthesis? Another word to make me feel stupid?"

"It's an upper-extremity prosthetic device that works off muscle feedback. It's a miracle for those who can work with it. However, not everyone is a candidate for this device."

"I am," I said.

"They told me that there's another course starting in a month. I'll find out if you can attend. I think it would be a good thing for you. Now, why don't you get some rest."

"There's plenty of room in this bed, Marly—are you tired?"

She smiled as she left the room.

I closed my eyes and began thinking about going home. I thought about what Marly had said about my parents picking me up. Suddenly I had a gnawing feeling in my gut that was all too familiar. Anxiety replaced my joy. Would my parents be there? Would they remember, or would they let other "activities" deplete their memory banks? I had spent a whole lifetime being disappointed by them. Why would tomorrow be any different?

I closed my eyes and suddenly saw myself as a nine-year-old child standing in front of the school. Football practice was over and all the parents were picking up their sons. Well, *almost* all. There was one conspicuous absence. I saw a sea of waving hands as they bade me farewell. I sat down on the bench as the knot in my stomach grew more noticeable. Nobody was coming to get me. Clouds began to gather over my head. "I'd better get home before I get caught in a downpour." And so, I started the long, lonely walk home. I knew that, upon entering the house, I would be greeted with apologies. It would be small consolation. It was not the first time it had happened, and "I'm sorry" had never taken away the pain in my gut.

CHAPTER 10

WAS AWAKENED FROM MY SLUMBER by the sound of
things being moved in my room. I opened my eyes
and saw that a staff nurse was placing my belongings
in a plastic bag.

"Let's get moving, Tony. There's a line waiting for
your bed. You have no idea what a popular place this is."

"It's probably because of Marly." I yawned.

"Marly? What's she got to do with it?"

"Never mind."

I was wheeled to the waiting room.

"Your parents will be here within the hour."

The anxiety was back. I hadn't seen my mother since
the accident. Occasionally my father had made some lame
excuse for why Mom could not come to visit me. It al-

ways reverted to how much she loved me and how she would be too upset to see me in my present condition. She never even called me. But, then again, Dad had an excuse for that. He told me that she was afraid that she would cry and upset me.

So I sat there, staring at the big wall clock.

Even the clock has two hands, I thought. But why were they moving so slowly?

"Excuse me." I got the attention of a woman with a broom. "Is that clock broken?"

"Nope. It might be a couple of minutes slow, but it's working."

An hour passed, and my parents were still not there. I closed my eyes and tried to imagine them walking through the doorway.

"This way, ma'am."

I looked up and saw my mom coming towards me. I wanted to hug her but I was paralyzed with anger.

"Sorry I'm late. This hospital is so confusing, and nobody gives you proper directions. Meanwhile, I'm missing *All My Children.*"

"How about *this* child, Mom? Did you miss me, too? Did you notice I've been gone? Did you hear that I'm missing one of my arms?" I waved my stump at her.

She looked away. "I heard all about it. Don't worry,

Tony, they have wonderful artificial parts these days."

Suddenly she leaned down and gave me a big hug. I looked into her eyes. They were red, and I realized she had been crying. "I'm sorry that I haven't been to see you. It's just very painful for me."

"I know." Once again I felt as if I were comforting my mother instead of the other way around. "Let's go home. What happened to my apartment?"

"Oh, Tony, we had to get rid of it. We couldn't keep paying rent while you weren't there. Don't worry, your friends packed up all your stuff and took it to our house. There's no way you can live by yourself. You'll need someone to take care of you."

The words sounded foreign coming from her mouth. I was having a difficult time recalling any time that she had ever taken care of me. On the other hand (no pun intended), there were countless nights when I had taken care of her. A vision of her lying on the floor passed through my mind. I blinked to clear it away.

"That will be great, Mom. I understand that a nurse will be coming to the house three times a week."

CHAPTER 11

MARLY WAS TRUE TO HER WORD, and a couple of short days after I returned home, my bell rang. I couldn't wait to open the door and see the lovely lady who would be tending to my wounds.

A corpulent woman stood on the other side of the door. It certainly wasn't Marly. In fact, it looked more like Harley. "You must be the patient."

Very observant, I thought. Did she think the wheelchair was a recreational vehicle? "Yes, that's me. Although I've been known to be impatient."

"I heard that you had a good sense of humor. Too bad you didn't have the sense to stay off the State Thruway on your bike."

This woman knew all about me.

"Well, let's get busy. We want to get you out and about, don't we? . . . I am going to dress your arm and leg."

She went about her business demonstrating the meaning of the word "efficient."

"See you on Thursday," she bellowed as she prepared to leave.

Twice a week, I was treated to the expertise of Nurse Harley, whose real name was Nurse Stone. Each time she left, I would remember the course Marly had told me about.

The following visit, I remembered to ask her while she was still within hearing distance.

"What did you say? Course?"

"Yes. Did Marley ever mention a course that she wanted me to attend?"

"Nope, can't say that she did, but I have a lot on my mind. I'll ask her when we discuss your case. Everyone is very excited at how miraculously you've been doing."

I had become, not only the embodiment of determination, but the topic of discussion. "I am fine" had become my mantra. "I can walk." I repeated those words over and over again as I did the strengthening exercises. Maybe there was something to this business about the power of positive thinking. In any event, it was worth a try. My inner dialogue was never silent. And, after two short weeks, a real miracle happened. I took my first step. Nurse Stone actually squealed with delight.

"Tony, I am so proud of you."

"I walked." I repeated the statement over and over again as if I had done something that nobody had ever, prior to that moment, accomplished. Then I literally hugged my legs and wept.

"Thank you, God," I said out loud, surprising myself with this sudden religious exclamation.

The nurse looked quietly at me.

"They say you don't appreciate something until you lose it, eh, Nurse Stone?

"Yes, Tony. I have had my share of losses in life. You have to make every moment count."

Suddenly I felt as if Chip were back. I thought of the wisdom that he had shared with me in what seemed like lifetimes ago. I thought about all the wasted time I'd spent being a know it all and a big shot. I thought of all the scamming I had done. Suddenly I felt ashamed.

"Nurse, maybe I don't deserve to walk." I had voiced my innermost fear.

"Now, you cut that out." Nurse Stone frowned at me. "We have all done things which we regret. Let's not look back—it will not serve you in the least."

"I have a favor to ask, Nurse Stone. Could I be transferred to the outpatient unit for therapy?"

"I don't see why not. Let me check with the rest of the staff."

IT SEEMED LIKE AN ETERNITY until Nurse Stone reappeared for her next scheduled visit. And when she did, she was wearing the biggest grin I had ever seen. "Tony, you are going to be doing your rehabilitation at the outpatient unit. Your progress has astounded everyone."

"Even me," I responded. "Thank you."

CHAPTER 12

ONE OF THE HAPPIEST DAYS of my life was when I drove myself to the Outpatient Unit. I was quite a celebrity. Everyone made a fuss over me and Marley even gave me a hug. "It's the amazing, Mr. T." It was better than balloons.

"By the way, Marley, whatever happened to that course you had mentioned, the one you wanted me to take?"

"Nurse Stone didn't tell you about it?" Marley looked upset. "I told her, but I guess she forgot to mention it. We have been so short-staffed with the budget cuts."

"What's the verdict?"

"Well." Marly smiled mysteriously. "They contacted me, and they not only want you to attend, but they need a patient model. And here's the best part yet. They are willing to pay you a hundred dollars if you'll accept."

"If I *accept?* Are you *kidding?* Of course I accept—my mind is still functioning. Marly, can I jump for joy?"

"Tony, do me a favor and wait a few weeks before you start jumping."

CHAPTER 13

THE COURSE WAS ALL I HAD HOPED FOR and more. Until that point I had not realized how isolated I felt. I had been a partial person in a world filled with whole people. But here, in this room, I was one of many with similar disabilities. We shared our histories, our fears, and our pain. It was like a family. In fact, it was like the family I had never had.

The course was conducted by a sales representative and an occupational therapist. As I watched the presentation, a thought occurred to me: *This demonstration would have been a lot more effective if the sales rep had been an amputee.*

Suddenly a bulb went off in my brain, and my imagination began painting pictures in front of me. I could see myself standing in front of the room.

Yes, I thought, if anyone were giving this course, it should be me.

At that point I realized that, one day, it *would* be me!

The next scene of my life was rapidly unfolding, and I was struggling to keep up with the momentum.

You see, at that very moment I knew I was going to become a sales representative. Not only would I, but my presentation would have a much greater impact than what I was hearing from the man standing in front of me. My presentation would be more effective because I would be wearing a company-provided prosthetic device.

I once again envisioned myself addressing an audience. As they listened to me, they were mesmerized. All through the talk, I'd keep the focus on my biological hand. And then, as the talk was ending, I would floor the audience by showing them that I was wearing the myo-electric prosthesis.

A vision of a man across the room snapped me out of my daydream. He was an upper-extremity amputee like myself. But, unlike me, he was wearing the myo-electric hand.

I began studying the people in the room. There was a guy who was missing both hands and both legs, yet he was standing by the wall. It was his prosthetic devices that enabled him to stand.

Sitting to my left was a guy busily writing. I was surprised to see that he too was wearing a prosthetic device. I began studying the contents of his paper. Using the device, he was drawing geometric figures. I couldn't believe how precise they were. He saw me staring.

"Hi," he whispered. "My name is Edmund. It's pretty amazing what these devices can do, isn't it?"

"It's unbelievable."

"Don't worry, you'll be able to do the same thing and a lot more."

The presenter called Edmund to the front of the group, where he told his story and showed his audience the drawings.

After that, they called me to come forward. The occupational therapist told me that he was going to do an evaluation. My heart pounded.

They placed myo-electrodes on my forearm to see if I could send a proper signal to a computer, which displayed a virtual prosthetic hand.

Much to my delight, I was able to control the hand on the computer.

"Great work. You picked this up really quickly," the OT exclaimed.

Then she turned to the group.

"Don't always expect to see such a positive demonstration. This young man is quite exceptional. It usually takes a long time to build the muscles in the residual limb. Congratulations, Mr. Risoli—you are an excellent candidate for a myo-electric prosthetic device."

I breathed a sigh of relief. Another obstacle had been removed from my path. However, my joy was short lived.

How would I pay for the hand? During the presentation, I had heard the sales rep say that the hand cost over $30,000.00. I approached Edmund. "I hope you don't mind if I ask you a personal question."

"Go right ahead."

"These hands are very expensive. How did you pay for yours?"

"Oh, that's easy," Edmund replied. "I had Medicaid pay for it."

". . .How do you get Medicaid?"

Edmund asked, "How much money do your parents make?"

"Not much. I've always had financial aid in school."

"Oh, then you shouldn't worry at all. I'm sure you'll meet the criteria. Just go to your local Department of Social Services and apply. Nothing to it, except for having to get up very early. After you get the Medicaid, give me a call, and I'll tell you what documents you need to get them to pay for the device."

Edmund and I continued to talk. He informed me that one of his prosthetists had made the arm in Brooklyn. He wrote down the man's name and phone number. "He'll be a great ally in your fight with Medicaid."

Next I approached the sales rep. I wanted to find out how he had gotten the job, so I could emulate him.

"What do I have to do to be you?"

"Go to school and get your degree in Communication. Then give me a call."

CHAPTER 14

I CAME HOME FEELING AN INCREDIBLE sense of peace. If anyone had asked, I would have said that I had a guardian angel. Things were falling into place. I had a plan.

The next day I went back to the junior college where i had gotten my associates degree. I enrolled in a marketing class. It was important for me to experience what it felt like being one-handed in a school environment.

The teacher was very understanding as we conferred. He said that he understood my situation, and that I need not worry if I had to skip classes for doctor's appointments; after all, the grade was irrelevant.

My next step was to file for Medicaid. I knew exactly what documents to bring to the Medicaid office, because, sadly, I had seen my mother do it more times than I care dto admit. However, I was not as fortunate as she had been. I got denied.

After that, I applied for Social Security Disability. This too turned out to be a disappointment. It was time to call Edmund.

"You live in a small suburb, right?" Edmund had the answer. "I heard that Social Services in the city is a lot more lenient. Maybe you should live there."

The city? It had always been my dream to live there. In my mind, it was a magical place filled with energy and nightlife. I obsessed about it for days. Maybe it was time to make this dream come true.

The following day, I ran into an ex-teacher of mine. We had always had a great relationship.

"Anthony! I cannot believe my eyes. You look wonderful."

"Thanks, Mrs. Sherman."

She gave me a big hug.

"Oh, Anthony, I am so sorry about your accident. I have been wondering how you are doing. But now that I see you, I must say that you look great. How are you making out, and what brings you back to our fair college?"

I explained why I felt a need to experience a classroom

now that I had a disability. I was "testing the waters." "I have plans, Mrs. Sherman—I want to get a degree in communications and become a prosthetic salesman."

"You are quite a young man. I have no doubt that you are going to realize your goals. I'm really impressed, Anthony. I always knew that you had a good head on your shoulders. Now I see that you have a very special quality."

"The question is, where should I go to finish my bachelor's? Before my accident, my plans were pretty well set. I was going to go to Florida. But now all that has changed. I don't really feel like being on a beach with my arm missing."

"Have you ever heard of Hoover College in the city? I understand they have an excellent communications program, and it's a CUNY school. In other words, it is relatively inexpensive for a four-year college. I bet your financial aide would cover it."

Was this another chance meeting? Was it an accidental conversation? No, I didn't believe so. Maybe there wasn't anything random about these events. They almost felt as if they were destined to happen. Was I the one who was making the plans, or was there a greater power at work? I didn't really know the answer. All I knew was that I felt extremely grateful.

Now, all I had to do was find a way to move to the city and be in Hoover College by January.

CHAPTER 15

L IVING WITH MY PARENTS FELT like a giant step backwards. It was stressful. There was constant friction in the house, and it brought back all the memories of my childhood and how miserable I had been there. All I could think about was the city and Hoover College. It was time to tell my parents about my future plans.

I sat down with my mom while my father lay behind us on the couch, his eyes glued to the television.

"Mom, I'm going to go to Hoover College in the city."

". . .What? How are you going to pay for that, or are you expecting your father and me to support you forever?"

"No, I'm going to get an apartment in the city and get

financial assistance."

"Tony, you're being ridiculous. The city is really expensive—have you checked it out? You're living rent free in this house. If you ask me, you have a great deal."

"Mom, I have all the furniture from my last apartment, so that's one big expense I don't have to worry about. And I also should have some spare cash. I saved a lot of money from all my part-time jobs."

My father decided that our conversation was more interesting than his television show. "Tony, your furniture is gone. The U-Haul we'd rented wasn't big enough, so we had to get rid of most of it."

". . .You got rid of my *stuff?*" I couldn't believe what I was hearing. "I worked hard to buy those things. How about my cash?"

"How did you think we were going to pay for the U-Haul? They don't give those away, you know. We had to rent it and put gas in the tank."

His voice sounded as if even he didn't believe the yarn he was spinning. "Tony, the electric bill was a little higher than we'd thought, so we took some more of that money to pay it. You understand."

No, I did not understand. I never had understood. This was a replay of a scene that had occurred over and over again. My parents routinely asked to borrow twenty dollars, but they never really knew the meaning of the word "borrow." In my dictionary, a loan gets repaid. In theirs, a loan becomes a gift.

"Look, Tony, we're offering you a chance to live here. Why must you be so ungrateful?"

"Thanks, anyway, Dad." I was too upset to argue. "I have made up my mind. I want to go to college in the city, and I want to live there."

"OK" Dad put on his jacket. "By the way, Tony, could I borrow a twenty? I'm out of beer and burgers. and tonight looks like a great night to barbeque."

"Sure, Dad. Enjoy yourself. Before you go, could you tell me where the remainder of my things are?"

"Sure. They're in the closet under the basement steps."

Under the basement steps. I couldn't believe my ears. How could all my stuff fit into that small space?

When I entered the closet, I found the answer to my question. Most of my things were gone. I no longer had a bed, a television, a microwave, and lots of my clothing. Had I supplied the merchandise for a garage sale as I lay in a coma? I looked nervously at the metal box in the corner. That was where I had stored my cash.

When I began working, my parents had advised me against bank accounts. They'd explained that the government knew every move you made when you kept your money in a bank. If you kept it in your home, nobody was the wiser.

Later on the lesson became clearer. I learned that it was very helpful to have "financial secrets" when applying for "financial aid."

A lump appeared in my throat as I opened the metal box. My eyes caught sight of a piece of paper on which I had scrawled *9,000 bucks.*"

I could not imagine how much my parents had "borrowed," so I decided to count what was there. It certainly didn't feel like $9,000.00 dollars to me, but maybe I was not aware of what $9,000.00 dollars felt like.

When I finished adding the bills, my stash had been reduced to $6,000.00. I counted again. The lump had moved to my chest. Three thousand dollars of my hard-earned money had been "borrowed."

I ran upstairs and started screaming at my mother. Dad came in the door carrying his beer and chopped meat. "You were stealing my savings while I was lying in a fucking coma?"

"Take it easy, Tony—we needed to pay the mortgage. You know this is your house, too."

I stood there shaking my head from side to side. Words failed me.

"Tony, business has really been slow. It's hard to support a family, but you wouldn't know about that kind of responsibility. Also, I was going to the hospital every day to see you. Do you know how expensive gas and tolls are?"

Oh, sure. It was my fault. My head started pounding. I wanted to run out of the house. I wanted to curse them. Instead, I ran up to my room. A temper tantrum was not going to help. I needed to get out of the insane asylum, and I needed to do it quickly.

The next day, I skipped classes and headed to the city. It was as if I were back in middle school, cutting classes and setting out on an adventure.

CHAPTER 16

GOT OFF THE COMMUTER BUS and headed to a news stand. "It shouldn't be difficult to find an apartment in this big city," I murmured to myself. I looked at some of the listings. They were worse than I thought. The rents seemed astronomical. Perhaps I should get the help of a realtor.

Things were even worse at the realtor's office. When I told him what I wanted to spend, he actually laughed at me. "You don't know this place, do you, young man? What you are looking at will cost you at least $3,000.00, plus our realtor's fee."

"Well, I'm glad I gave you a laugh," I barked as I stormed out of his office. However, I knew that it wasn't the man's fault. I was a clueless kid from the suburbs. He probably wasn't trying to be mean. It's just that I felt so vulnerable. But I had no intentions of crawling back to my parents on my hands and knees and admitting defeat.

I returned home. Tomorrow would be another day and another search.

The following day, I headed back to the city, but, this time, I went downtown to a neighborhood I'd explored in my youth. I purchased a local paper.

For Rent By Owner, read the headline. The price was $1,100.00. "Wow. It's near Jefferson Park. That's a fun area."

I called the number in the newspaper.

"Hello, this is Monica. May I help you?"

She sounded elderly. "Yes, ma'am. I saw your ad for an apartment in the *Jefferson Review.* Could I see it?"

"You're lucky to catch me in. I'm showing the place at three o'clock. It's a really big room. I'm sure it will go very quickly. But if you don't get that apartment, I have a place not far way that's only $900.00 a month. It's a little smaller but great for a single person."

She gave me the address and directions on how to get there. They seemed simple enough, but as I followed them, I realized that the blocks were much longer than I'd realized. I stared nervously at my watch as the big hand crept over the numbers. Oh, no, I thought. By the time I get to that apartment, Monica will probably be shaking the hand of her new tenant, and it won't be me. I broke into a run and reached my destination breathless as my watch displayed 3:10 on its face.

"Hi," I panted. "I'm Tony."

"Tony, I am so sorry, but I told you that the apartment would probably be grabbed up immediately. The first man who came here fell in love with the place. In fact, he was so enthusiastic that he got here before I did. But don't be upset—I told you that I have another apartment for rent. Wanna see it now?"

"The smaller one?"

"Don't jump to conclusions. It's not that small, and you're not that big." She laughed. "We can walk there— it's only two blocks from here."

We walked along together like old friends. There was something I liked about Monica. She seemed so warm and caring; like the grandmother I had never had.

"So tell me, Tony, what happened to your arm? Were you born that way?"

"No, ma'am, I was in a motorcycle accident." The last thing I felt like doing was discussing my story, but I did not want to appear rude.

She seemed to sense my hesitancy and changed the subject. "How are you planning on paying for the apartment?

"I'm starting a new job next week. In the meantime, I have savings that I can use."

"You seem like a very nice young man. I like a person who saves and plans for things. So many of the young people these days don't know the value of a dollar. I have been showing apartments for quite some time, and you can't believe the people I've met. Bums, drug addicts, you name it. . . . You don't do drugs, do you, Anthony?"

"Of course not. I have plans ,and drugs are not a part of them."

"You're not only good-looking, but you're smart. I like that. You know, I'm a good judge of character."

She paused in front of a small building. "Here she is."

I glanced around at the neighboring stores. Across the street sat a falafel place. My mouth began to water. There were hip-looking shops and, on the corner, a bar. I was falling in love.

"This looks like a great block."

"Let's see the apartment now. Sorry, Tony, but there's no elevator in this building. I hope you don't mind a little walk, you know it's good for your heart."

." . .What floor is it on?"

"It's on the fourth floor, and if I can do it, you can do it."

"No problem."

The steps were steep but I didn't mind.

"Don't tell me you're out of breath!"

"No," I replied. "I am just so excited about seeing the place."

Monica pointed to a door at the end of the hall. "That's the bathroom. Let's have a look."

It seemed adequate to me. It had a shower, a bowl and a sink. "Whose bathroom is it?" I asked.

"It's the bathroom for the apartment you are about to see. I hope you don't mind that it's down the hall."

"Do I have to share it with anyone?"

"Nope, it's all yours. You can even put a lock on the door, as long as you give me a spare key. Fire regulations, you know."

"Let's have a look at the room."

She inserted her key in the lock, and the door squeaked its welcome.

I looked around at my possible new "crib." The floors were covered with linoleum that was a bit ripped in places. The refrigerator was small, but, then again, so was the whole place. I walked over to the window at the rear of the room to check the view. It looked out on an alley that was gradually being turned into a garbage dump.

It did not qualify as a view. "Eyesore" was more appropriate.

She saw me staring. "People are such slobs. So, what do you think? Are you interested?"

"Yes." I fell over my words.

"Then it's yours. OK?"

"OK."

"It will be $2,700.00, which takes care of two months' rent and a month's security. I hope you have that much in savings."

"I do."

"Then we're going to have to go through some standard lease agreements. And, of course, I will need a deposit." She took a sheet of paper from her folder.

"Would you mind if I took the lease home and read it carefully? It's getting sort of late, and I have to catch a bus. I'll call you early tomorrow. "

"No problem, Tony. It's just a standard lease agreement. But would you mind leaving a deposit?"

"I have $200.00. Is that OK?"

"Sure." She scribbled a receipt for the deposit. "It's refundable in case something comes up."

"Bye, now, Monica. Thanks!"

"It was a pleasure meeting you. And, by the way, I think you will be very happy in this place."

CHAPTER 17

THAT NIGHT I SHOWED MY PARENTS the lease. "This is pretty routine—it looks good to me," my father commented. "How did you get such a cheap place? Does it have a roof?"

"Yes, I'll be sleeping on it. I sure could have used that couch that you—ahem—couldn't fit in the U-Haul."

Mom made another attempt to tighten the umbilical chord. "I don't understand why you're moving to that dirty city. It's so beautiful here. Why don't you drop this ridiculous idea?"

I looked at her and shook my head. There was no need for words.

The next morning, I called Monica early. "When can I take the place?"

"Sorry, Tony, but it won't be ready until the first of the month. I have to paint it and spruce it up. You deserve a nice clean place, don't you?"

I was overjoyed. The extra time would give me a chance to get a job and to apply to Hoover.

"Can I meet with you on Monday next week? I have an appointment with the admissions counselor at Hoover College, so I can drop off the lease and the money."

"Sounds good. See you then."

That weekend, I spent making lists. I had to figure out how much money I would need to cover my expenses in my new crib as well as what furniture and utensils I would have to purchase.

My mother walked into my room. "If you want to take some dishes and silverware, you can. I also have extra towels." She was trying to appear jolly, but I could see the sadness in her eyes. "Tony, I'm sorry that I've given you such a hard time. I love you."

"I love you too, Mom. And. . .thanks."

"Tony, one more thing—will you be home for holidays?"

"Of course." I smiled and hugged her.

Not only had she offered to help, but my friends, upon hearing about my new place, also said they would be of assistance, too.

"Anything you need, Tony, just ask."

"Do you need me to help you bring your stuff to the city?"

I felt truly grateful to have so many loyal friends. But a lot of the things that needed to be done were solo jobs. My head was already swimming. First of all, I needed to tell the community college that I'd be leaving.

I approached my college professor and let him know my change of plans. He was very supportive and wished me well in my new career path.

THE DAY I HAD BEEN WAITING FOR finally arrived, and I headed nervously to the city to meet with the administrator at Hoover College. I had given myself plenty of time and, as I strolled leisurely down the street, my eyes glanced at my new neighborhood.

"Got a quarter, pal?" A homeless man walked in front of me.

I fumbled with the change in my pocket. "Sure."

I looked around and noticed what appeared to me as a lot of homeless people begging for money. Would I be safe in this neighborhood? I was a young suburban kid, a bit shocked by what I was seeing. I wondered what the streets would be like late at night.

Of course I'd be safe, I consoled myself. After all, I'd

been through, I was not going to let some beggars stop me from realizing my dreams.

As I approached Hoover College, the homeless people slipped out of view and out of my mind. Fear was replaced by excitement.

A sign clearly pointed the way to the administrative office. "Sign in, please," said a cheerful receptionist, who smiled at me.

I looked around. It reminded me of a doctor's waiting room. There were at least twenty people sitting and squirming. I found an empty seat and joined them.

Finally my name was called, and I met with a friendly young man. "Tony Risoli, I'm Steve Summers. Have a seat." I noticed how he gave a quick glance at my missing limb. "What degree are you pursuing?"

"I have a Marketing associate's degree, but I'd like to shift into Corporate Communications. "

"That sounds great. Hoover welcomes students who know what they want. Goals are important and, these days, so few young people have them. We have to see which of your past courses will roll over into this program."

Another hour later, I had my classes picked out, had obtained financial aid, and was another step closer to my all-important goal.

I left the college feeling upbeat. Did the neighborhood look less forbidding, or was I just trying to reassure myself? The one thing that bothered me was the time slot of the Mandated Psychology course. It finished at 10:00 p.m. I visualized myself walking through the streets in the dark and recalled my dream of homeless people falling out of doorways.

"Enough of this!" I said out loud. I could not allow fear any space in my day. I had too much to accomplish.

I looked at my watch. *Oh, no!* I was late for my appointment with Monica.

I practically flew down the subway steps and grabbed the Number 7 train. My adolescent sojourns into the city had once again come in handy, and I was quite familiar with the subway system. I thought back to that young boy fearlessly exploring the city. I was fearless then, and I would be fearless now.

I got to Monica's breathless and only ten minutes late. "You're late again, Tony," she said. That's a bad quality." She was carrying a briefcase in one hand and a cell phone in the other. "If you'd come a minute later, I'd have been gone. This is a business I'm running, and time is money. I told you that you were very lucky to get that apartment. It's a steal. I probably could have gotten more money for it if I'd held out. However, we'd made a deal and I always keep my word. Do you have the papers and the money?"

I tried to ignore her attitude, but I must admit I was angry. This woman is not going to step all over me, I thought. I wanted to tell her to fuck herself, and that the deal was off. But, instead, I smiled politely and handed her the papers. Thank God I was learning some self-control.

I left her with a sinking feeling in my gut. Was this any indication of the kind of landlady she was going to be?

"Can I have a dollar for a cup of coffee?" A disheveled man was looking sadly at me once I was back on the street.

"Leave me alone!" I snapped. I pushed my stump in his face. "See this? You have two arms. Get yourself a job."

I wasn't proud of myself for taking out my frustration on that unfortunate soul, but I was feeling tense.

Had I said "job"? I'd almost forgotten. *I* was the one who needed to get a job. After all, my savings were quickly dwindling, and Monica obviously wasn't going to let me live rent-free. It was time to do some serious thinking.

My last job had been as a catering coordinator, and I had enjoyed it very much. I remembered that they had a branch in the city. Perhaps it was time to give my former boss a call.

"Hi, Mr. Giacono. This is Tony Risoli."

"Anthony! It's so great to hear from you. How are you making out?"

All he had to do was ask. I went into great detail about my plans, and how I had one missing link. . .a job. "Didn't you once tell me that Catering Needs had a branch in the city?"

"Yes, it has a big branch there. You want me to call the sales manager, Bob Harris, and see if he needs some help?"

"That would be great, Mr. G.!"

"I'm sure that he can use you—he needs hard workers. And he'll be even more likely to hire you when I tell him what a good worker you were. Would you like me to call him now?"

"*Yes!*" I practically yelled into the phone. "Could you get back to me as soon as you speak with him?"

"Sure, Tony. You were like a son to me. It would be my pleasure to help you out."

Not only did he speak to Bob Harris, he faxed my resume and references to him.

A little over an hour later, he called back. "Bob seemed impressed," he told me. "Unfortunately, he's not sure when a position will be opening, but let's keep our fingers crossed. There's someone presently on his staff that he might have to let go. If you don't hear from him in a couple of weeks, give him a call. He'll like your enthusiasm."

I was a little disappointed but determined to keep hope alive.

After all, positive thinking had been paying off so far.

By the time I boarded the bus back to suburbia, I had an apartment, my college courses in place, and the prospect of a job at Catering Needs.

CHAPTER 18

MOVING WAS TOUGHER than I had imagined. Rob drove his van, and we piled my few meager belongings inside. Kyle's parents had donated a sleep sofa and a dresser to their favorite charity—me.

The traffic was impossible as Rob navigated the van into the city, cursing all the way. "Is it always rush hour here?" he grumbled.

Finally, after an hour's worth of irritation, we pulled up in front of the apartment building. "Is there an elevator?" he asked.

"Are you serious? It's a fourth-floor walk-up."

"Oh, that will be fun. I can see us dragging your stuff up the flights." Kyle clutched at his heart.

As we started unloading the van, the door to the building opened, and a guy covered with tattoos and piercings came out.

"Is that one of your neighbors?" Rob and Kyle were laughing.

"Don't be so judgmental, man." I was feeling annoyed but didn't want to seem ungrateful after the grueling trip and what promised to be a hellish ascent up the staircases. For the first time, I was glad that my parents had gotten rid of much of my stuff. We were exhausted by the time we lugged up the last carton. "Where's the rest of your apartment?" Rob laughed.

I was getting more and more infuriated. Sure, it was no palatial estate, but I was trying to make the best of the situation.

"I need to use the bathroom," said Kyle. "Where is it?"

"At the end of the hall."

"You're kidding. You have to go out into the hall to take a crap?"

"It's only a short distance, man."

"Are you going to be sharing the bathroom with the tattooed man?"

"Not at all. Monica said that it's private, and I can put a lock on the door. . . . Hey, I'm getting sick of your wisecracks. This is my new home."

Rob looked serious. "Tony, are you sure you are not making a mistake? You had a really nice, big basement at your parents'."

The problem was that Rob was voicing my own insecurities. I didn't want to consider the possibility that the whole move had been a colossal error.

"Are you going to feed us?" Kyle asked.

"Sure. This neighborhood is crawling with restaurants."

"Yes, but are the restaurants crawling, too?"

I realized I was going to have to put up with those clowns and stop being so sensitive. We walked across the street to a Mexican restaurant.

"This looks like a nice place. Are you in the mood for Mexican food? If not, there's an Italian place down the corner."

"Italian food sounds good to me," Kyle said.

"And *there's* dessert," Rob said pointing at an ice cream parlor across the street.

Two attractive-looking girls were standing in front of the shop, enjoying their cones.

"Yes. That looks like a very fine dessert." Kyle stared at the lovelies.

"You know, T., this might not have been such a bad

move. This neighborhood is alive."

After stuffing ourselves, we hiked up the stairs to my place again, where we spent the remainder of our time trying to create a semblance of order.

"It's getting late, and I'm exhausted." Rob wanted to head back to the suburbs. "Enjoy your first night in paradise."

I said, "Thanks for everything," and meant it.

I plopped down on the sofa and closed my eyes. But even though I was totally wiped out, the noise in the street was distracting. How would I be able to sleep with that racket?

Oh, well, I concluded. If you can't beat them. . . . I grabbed my jacket and headed downstairs.

Maybe I'll go in for a beer, I thought. And then I thought twice. I was still underage and would be for another five months. How depressing. I looked into of a bar window; the place seemed to be filled with happy people. It looked so inviting—yet it was not inviting me inside, not for another five months.

A guy passed me and looked at my missing arm. "What's the matter, pal? Can you use a hand?"

"No thanks, I already have one." I was used to jokers like that. "Yes. Get me into that bar, *pal*."

". . .Actually, that's something I *can* do that for you.

Do you want me to make you a fake I.D.?"

"No, thanks. I'm OK." I was hoping I had left my shady ways in the suburbs.

Suddenly I was overwhelmed with fatigue. I climbed the stairs and lay back down on the sofa. Surprisingly, I could not hear the noise from the street anymore. All I could hear was the sound of my own snoring.

THE MORNING SUN ON MY FACE WOKE me up from a delicious sleep.

I'll have to get some curtains, I thought. This was where Mom would come in handy.

I thought about all the things I still had to do. Though I had some time before school began, I had not even begun to tackle the Medicaid office. I only hoped that Edmund had been right. The last thing I needed was a refusal.

In the beginning, it had been kind of special having one hand. But now I had grown thoroughly tired of that and was overcome by a sense of urgency. Medicaid equaled a prosthetic device.

Finding the Department of Social Services was a piece of cake for a city boy. Finding it half empty was even more of a blessing.

"Yes, I can help you." The man behind the counter looked tired, or was it bored?

I told him my story.

"That's quite a tale, Tony. You're pretty remarkable. I've have seen a lot of people sink under lighter weights, believe me. I'll speed up your process. Give me two weeks, and you will be the proud possessor of Medicaid."

Proud? I thought. My family had never seemed proud leaving Social Services in the suburbs.

Then it was time to call Edmund's prosthetist. I explained to him how I had met Edmund and how impressed I had been with his prosthetic. I told him that I had Medicaid on the way, and we set up an appointment.

He said, "It's a bit of a journey from where you are, Mr. Risoli. I hope you know the subway system. It can get a bit confusing when you have to transfer trains."

"No problem. Just give me the directions and an appointment."

"We're located in the third borough outside the city. Grab a pencil, and I'll tell you which trains to take." He gave me the address and some directions that sounded as if they were in a foreign language.

"It shouldn't be difficult," I said. "I have subway maps in my room."

"It's about a forty-five-minute trip, so give yourself extra time. See you tomorrow bright and early."

That night I lay in bed tossing and turning. I was too

excited to drift easily into sleep. I kept thinking about how wonderful it would be to have two hands again. I felt grateful. I thought about Chip and how he had up-lifted my spirits when things felt so bleak. I thought about Edmund and how helpful he'd been. I thought about the nursing staff, even the difficult personalities. Just then, I loved every one of them, even Nurse Ratchet. They had all helped to bring me closer to my goal. I was going to be "complete" again. Finally, I couldn't fight it any longer, and sleep overcame me—and, along with it, dreams.

I was walking down the street, proudly displaying my new hand and forearm, but nobody seemed to be noticing. I was holding it in the air, but people kept passing me. I began taking quarters out of my pockets and giving them to derelicts, using my right hand. Some said, "Thank you." Some didn't say anything.

I finally said, "Look, I have a new hand."

"Nice, buddy," a bum acknowledged me.

"Thanks!" I was beaming.

THE BUZZER AWAKENED MY BLISS. I began to get ready for the long trip. I rolled my right sleeve down, covering up my missing limb. Perhaps this would be the last time I'd have to. The thought filled me with immeasurable joy.

I headed to the subway at 6:00 a.m. Yes, it seemed ridiculously early, but I wasn't going to take any chances of being late. The scene on the street distracted me. I saw people staggering, obviously drunk from their night of partying. Some were heading into the falafel place. I envied them. They looked so happy. How I would have loved to be part of the festivities, but I had more important things to do. I wiped any feelings of envy from my mental slate and descended into the subway.

Happily, the first train pulled in to the station as I arrived. According to Dr. Wegman, the prosthetist, I was supposed to be on train number one for approximately ten stops and get off at Jubilee Junction. I looked around the car. There were relatively few occupants, most of them dressed very nicely. I figured they were on their way to their respective offices. Someday, I would be doing the same.

A sitting mother was holding her child, who couldn't have been more than a year old. Was it my imagination, or was the kid staring at my empty sleeve? I was used to strange stares and uncomfortable glances. Sometimes young people would be more direct and ask me, "What happened to your arm?"

The train pulled into Jubilee Junction, a strange name for the stop: It was dark and dreary-looking. I was grateful that my next train arrived quickly. And yet, once on board, my feelings of gratitude turned to feelings of discomfort. The occupants were seedy. One guy had a radio blasting hip-hop. Another was sprawled out on the seat, sound asleep, disheveled, and there was a distinct odor coming from him. A mother had given up trying to control her child, and the child was climbing all over the car and kicking people.

"Want me to smack your little bastard?" a passenger yelled. "I already have a headache. *I'll* shut your kid up if you can't."

Suddenly, he turned to me. "Hey, look. There's a one-armed bandit."

I pretended I hadn't heard him. I pretended that I didn't see what was going on. I looked straight ahead. Dr. Wegman had told me that I'd be on this second train for about twenty-five minutes, and I was trying hard to avoid any altercations.

I breathed a sigh of relief when we pulled into the Q Street station.

My final train ride promised to be a quick one, although finding the right track was a bit confusing.

Another sleazy crowd: I looked around. At least this was going to be a short trip.

Dr. Wegman was a man of his word. I felt as if I had just boarded when the train pulled into the Brook Avenue station. My adventure was almost over, but I knew it was well worth it.

Dr. Wegman's office was only a block away from the subway, and I was right on time. "What an ordeal," I said to the receptionist as I signed in.

There were already two men sitting in the waiting room. This doctor doesn't waste anytime, I thought as I looked at the men. Both were missing a leg. They could make a matched set if they walked together, I laughed to myself.

The minute I met Dr. Wegman, I liked him. He possessed a well-honed bedside manner. Edmund had pretty much shared the details of my case, so I was spared going through the tedious story of the wheelies.

"It's going to be awhile before we get approval from Medicaid," he said, "and before you're ready for the prosthesis. In the meantime you will have to work with an occupational therapist to strengthen the residual limb.

"While you are doing that, I will be doing battle with the Medicaid Department. But don't worry, I am a master at it. You'll have to call and make an appointment with the occupational therapist. Your school is near Beldale Hospital, and they have a wonderful OT named Rosalie Burger. People call her Ms. Rosalie. You'll like her, Tony."

"How long will this process take?" I felt myself growing impatient.

"It should be about two months before I get the authorization. But relax, Tony. You'll really enjoy Ms. Rosalie, and you will be well-strengthened by then. At that point, you'll return to my office, so that I can cast your arm and make a socket."

"Ah, Marly, where are you now?"

"What was that?" Dr. Wegman looked at me suspiciously.

"Oh, nothing, I was just remembering a wonder OT I had, I mean for therapy."

As I left Dr. Wegman's, I glanced at my watch. It was already 8:30, and I had that endless trip home ahead of me. Yet I was filled with optimism. The two months would fly by, and I would be determinedly building my strength.

It was easy getting back to my apartment and I felt like a pro.

MY FRIEND SKIP WAS COMING to spend the day and night with me. He was an old friend from high school. His real name was Sam, but he'd earned the nickname "Skip" by his skillful art of skipping classes.

I had time for a short nap before the downstairs buzzer

awakened me. "Who is it?"

"Come on, man. Stop with the 'who is it' shit. Just buzz me up."

Skip began the climb.

"This is a cool neighborhood, T.," said he when he reached my floor. "I know it pretty well. Lots of bars around here, too."

"A lot of good they do me," I frowned. "I'm not quite at the age when I can drink legally. But I've only a few months left."

"A few *months?*" Skip was irritated. "I didn't come all the way in from the suburbs to sit in your spacious crib. Haven't you ever heard of fake I.D.'s?"

"Yes. When I first moved in, a guy approached me, trying to sell me one. I figured that I was so close to my birthday that I didn't want to risk it."

"Well, you are going to risk it today, my man. This is a great neighborhood, and we are going to take advantage of it."

Skip was two years older than I was, so he had nothing to worry about.

"Don't look so serious, T. Everybody does it. In fact, I know exactly where you can get a fake one." We walked a few blocks past Jefferson Park. Skip came to an abrupt stop in front of a place called Rusty's Smoke Shop.

"Ah, good old Rusty. This is an icon. My uncle even talked about it in the '80s. Rusty must be doing something right."

"Or wrong," I said. "Look, Skip, there's Vincent's Pizza Parlor. Everyone raves about their pies."

"Get your mind out of your stomach, T. We have important business to attend to." We entered the store.

I looked around at all the suspicious-looking pipes. I guess Rusty caters to the local weed crowd, I thought. Skip took charge as he approached the man behind the counter. "Listen, my man, this is my younger brother. He needs an I.D."

"For school?" The man winked. "Follow me." He led us to the back of the store and down a narrow flight of stairs to the basement.

Thirty minutes later, we resurfaced. I was staring at my first I.D. "Sweet." I was now John Dolan, official drinking dude.

"Let's celebrate at Joe's Caribbean," Skip suggested.

"I'm impressed, man. You certainly do know this hood."

"Let's say that I'm familiar with the important local spots."

Once inside Joe's, Skip and I got completely lost in a cloud of music and tequila and babes, babes, babes.

That night, Skip wound up staying with a girl whom he had met at the bar. I found my own female companion to share my bed, and, I must say, she was a lot easier on the eyes than Skip.

The next morning, I awakened with my head throbbing. I glanced over at the sleeping form stretched out beside me. Suddenly I felt a pang of remorse. I thought about my old girlfriend, Jenn, and all we had been through. It's never easy to say goodbye, but we'd felt it was best to go our separate ways when I moved to the city.

The buzzer pounded my already pounding head. It was the Prodigal Son returning.

"Tony, that was a helluva night. I hardly remember anything except, of course, Stephanie. Did you see that beauty? We are meeting later. You don't mind if I stay here for a few more days."

"No, not at all," I answered, looking at the sleeping Kathy.

FOUR DAYS LATER, AFTER NON-STOP PARTYING and Skip on my floor, reality pierced through the veil of booze. If I did not stop this, I would lose everything that I had worked so hard to acquire. School was starting the following week, and I had not even contacted Mr. Harris about the catering job.

"Skip! The party's over! Time for you to pack up and head back to the burbs."

"Oh, come on, T.—I have a date with Stephanie tonight."

"Then sleep at her place. Hotel Risoli is closed. The management will be attending school."

Skip whined a few more times. I reminded him that I did not have wealthy parents like he did. I reminded him that my parents did not take care of my financial needs. It was time for him to move on. "We'll do it again sometime."

I took the next couple of days to sober up and clear my head. Then I located my notebook and made one of my to-do lists. First on that list was a call to Mr. Harris of Catering Needs.

"Mr. Harris, this is Anthony Risoli, Mr. Giacono's friend. We spoke before."

"Of course, Tony, you saved me the trouble of a phone call. I have a spot opening up. Could you come in Monday for an orientation?"

"You bet!" I was back in the flow, and once more things were falling into place.

Next on my list was the Beldale Hospital and Ms. Rosalie.

"I would like to make an appointment with Rosalie

Burger."

"One moment, young man. Whom should I say is calling?"

"This is Anthony Risoli—Dr. Wegman referred me to Ms. Burger."

"Around here, she's known as Ms. Rosalie. But you'll get to know the drill. I'll connect you."

Ms. Rosalie and I talked for fifteen minutes and then set up an appointment for the first day of my classes. "Don't worry, Tony, we'll work around your school schedule. Bye, now."

Ms. Rosalie, I thought, placing the receiver in the cradle. Why does that name sound so familiar?

Suddenly it dawned on me. *Sister* Rosalie of Holy Saint!

I hadn't thought of that name for a long time. The infamous Sister Rosalie! Growing up I had heard stories she liked to give young boys "special attention" after their religion classes. It'd been one of those things people whispered and giggled about, but I'd never been sure if the stories were true.

Then one day, the day had come when I was finally enrolled in Sister Rosalie's religion class.

Here is my opportunity to experience the Sister's special tutorial, I thought.

But the day I arrived in her class had been the day of the her mysterious disappearance—and there, standing at the front of the room, had stood a Sister who looked more like a Mister. Sister Alex never strayed far from her ruler, her favorite weapon. Getting slammed on the knuckles was something to avoid, so her class sat at attention, hands folded. None of the students seemed to know what had happened to Sister Rosalie, and none had dared to ask.

I caught myself: Why was I thinking about the past? I had more important things to focus on than some sick suburban stories.

THE NIGHT BEFORE MY FIRST DAY OF CLASSES, I LAY in bed obsessing. How would I accomplish everything? I was starting school, occupational therapy, and orientation for my new job. Had I over committed myself?

Would they wind up committing me? It was a night of tossing and turning and listening to the laughter in the street. *Well, those carefree days are gone, T.* My thoughts waxed nostalgic.

It was time for a quick shower and getting ready to take on the day.

My first stop was Hoover College, where I spent a grueling three hours fighting to stay awake and to maintain the semblance of a positive outlook. It was the first time I'd willingly agreed to follow a mandated curriculum. No longer the boss of my life, I was playing by somebody else's rules. But I consoled myself with the realization that it was all a means to an end.

The school day climaxed with a monotonous lecture, and then I had to scurry over to see Ms. Rosalie. I hurried into Beldale Hospital, completed the registration, and headed to the Occupational Therapy Department.

"Glad to meet you, Tony." Ms. Rosalie picked up my spirits. She gave me a tour and told me how fortunate I was to be in the hospital. "We have state-of-the art equipment here."

After a rigorous workout, I left with my weekly follow-up schedule, which, as promised, fit neatly into my school curriculum. Onto the orientation session at Catering Needs!

I guess there'll be no time for lunch, I realized, my stomach growling. I'd better plan for this and bring something with me in the future.

Catering Needs was in a massive building on the east side of town—no dinky suburban operation.

Suburban Kid Hits Big Time. My mind was running wild with headlines.

"Hey, are you Anthony?" Mr. Harris asked by way of

greeting. I recognized his face from my googling experience on the Catering Needs website. "Follow me."

He led me to a room in which six other eager entries sat waiting. Next he placed a video tape into a player. "I shall return."

The tape began with the bold words *Orientation Training.* It was followed by a booming voice: *Here at Catering Needs, we cater to our customers first.*

From there on it was downhill. I knew all the information from my past experience and did not need the smiley faces and appetizing food staring at me. My stomach was screaming for something to eat; I felt like grabbing some *hors d'oeuvres* from the screen.

The video finally ended with a Catering Needs jingle, and Mr. Harris, right on cue, entered the room. Much to my horror, he popped in another video. "This is standard procedure, folks. Enjoy. Be sure to pick up your packets on the way out. And also, more importantly, be sure to read the contents. I'll be sending out our final work schedules by the end of the week. Welcome to the Tri City Mecca of Catering Needs, and glad to have you on board."

CHAPTER 19

ORKING WITH MS. ROSALIE and the occupational team, attending school, and going
to work proved to be quite doable and even,
I admit, enjoyable. It wasn't long before I could feel the
endurance building in my arm. My mind too was becoming stronger from all the information bombarding it. And
best of all, my wallet was growing thicker. Finally, I had
some cash to play with.

As I was sitting in the library, studying, my cell phone
rang.

"*Sh!*" a chorus of disgusted studiers chided me. Glanc-
ing down at the phone, I saw Dr. Wegman's number and
darted outside to accept the call.

"Well, it's all good, Tony. Medicaid has approved

your prosthesis, and we can start casting. I spoke with Ms. Rosalie, and she gave me a glowing report on your progress, so we're good to go. When can you come in?"

"I'll come in tomorrow, but I'm only available in the latter part of the afternoon."

"We can do that. Let me connect you with the receptionist."

We set up an appointment for 5:30 the following day.

The next day seemed insufferable. My eyes were focused on my watch as the hands dragged slowly around its face. My thoughts were focused on Dr. Wegman.

During occupational therapy, Ms. Rosalie sensed my anxiety. "What's the matter, Tony? Your mind seems to be elsewhere."

I told her about my appointment.

"Why don't you leave twenty minutes earlier today? It's a long trip out to the third borough. I got lost the first time I tried it."

"Thanks!" I darted out the door in search of the closest subway. This shouldn't be too complicated, I thought. I just had to add one more train connection, and I'd be on track. I smiled at my pun.

All was going smoothly until Jubilee Junction. Thank goodness for passers-by who willingly supplied directions. And thank goodness for Ms. Rosalie's twenty-minute gift.

I needed the extra time. When I finally got to Dr. Wegman's office, a packed waiting room greeted me.

"Sorry, Tony," the receptionist apologized. "We had an emergency, and the doctor is a bit backed up. Just pick up a magazine and relax."

An interesting magazine cover leapt out at me: *In Motion, From The Amputee Coalition of America.* It was great to see that there *was* such an organization helping amputees. My mind began its usual race as I opened the magazine. The thought of being part of such an organization flooded my brain.

Before I knew it, I was on the last page of the magazine. It was difficult to believe that I had read the whole thing. The clock looked down at me. Seven o'clock. An hour and a half had passed since I entered the waiting room. They don't call it a "waiting" room for nothing. I noticed that most of the people were gone, though. At least there was progress.

"Tony, you're next. That patient only needs a minor adjustment, so you'll be seeing the doctor within the next ten minutes."

The receptionist knew her timing, and ten minutes later, I was sitting with Dr. Wegman.

"All I really need is a cast of your arm. It should go quickly, Tony. I'm sorry you had such a long wait, but we had an emergency. Sometimes these things happen, but, thankfully, not very often."

As Dr. Wegman spoke, he took wet plaster strips and wrapped them around my stump. After he'd placed the twentieth strip on me, I could feel it hardening. "This is normal. We're almost finished."

Thirty minutes had passed; the clock read 7:45. I thought about the trains and wondered what the schedule would be like at such a late hour. Would the express trains still be running?

The mouth of the subway swallowed me up as I embarked on my long journey home. It had been an eventful day, and my mood was good despite the trip awaiting me.

But when I entered the belly of the beast, a disquieting feeling crept over me. Was it my imagination, or did the station have an ominous look, even more than usual? The platform was nearly deserted. "Come on Tony, snap out of it," said aloud. "You've been close to death. This is nothing."

I spotted a man sitting further down on the platform bench. It appeared to be an opportunity to find out about the train schedule. I went to join the stranger. But the closer I got, the stranger he looked. He was engaged in a heated discussion with the empty space next to him. I turned around and headed back to my original waiting area as a teenager snuck under the turnstile.

"Hi." I approached him. "I don't mean to scare you, but I'm new in the neighborhood. I've never been on this train at this hour. Does the express still run?"

"Can't you read?" He pointed to a sign. "The express trains stop running at 7:30. Enjoy your trip."

He turned his back on me.

I figured I would be seeing more tunnel scenery than I'd hoped, frustration building; but then I heard the welcome sound of a train heading my way.

"Take the last train to Clarksville," I began whistling.

The trip, despite its humble beginnings, was not as bad as my imagination had pictured. We screeched into Jubilee Junction soon enough. But as I disembarked, confusion greeted me. This platform was also fairly deserted, and I wondered whether my next train was running.

I saw two young guys standing in a huddle. One smiled at me through his missing teeth. "Lost, bro?"

"Yes, sort of. The trains don't seem to be running on schedule. I see that the R is running on the local track."

"Your problems are over, my man. Just follow us."

I looked at my escorts. What a motley crew—their pants were falling below their rears, and they had baseball caps on backwards. They're just kids, I told myself.

I noticed an angry-looking scar disfiguring one guy's

face and wondered what had caused it. It looked as if it still needed medical attention. Was I being paranoid? They're probably good kids, I kept reassuring myself. They looked about sixteen years old. Maybe, one day, I'll be able to do something worthwhile with this imagination, I concluded. "Right now, I am merely driving myself insane."

I followed them down to a corridor at the end of the platform. As we turned the corner, I could hear the sound of loud music. I seriously doubted that Jubilee Junction was supplying entertainment for its after-hours passengers.

At the turn, we were greeted by four older men. The smell of smoke hit me: definitely not tobacco. Two guys were was seated on a crate. One was wearing a white tank top. Seated next to him, his pock-marked companion was blasting a radio. The two other guys were standing and sneering at me.

"Hey, Ralphie—" the smoker got up and stamped out his joint. "You bring us a present?"

"He's lost," Ralphie told him. "Shall we help him?"

The radio went off. "Hey, look! He only has one arm. Ralphie, why did you bring us a gimp?"

"Listen, guys," I said, pretending I wasn't terrified. "I'm lost. I'm just trying to get back to the city. I lost my arm in a motorcycle accident."

"A motorcycle, huh? Expensive one? You some rich kid from the city?"

"No, I'm not rich at all."

"Liar! You probably live in some fancy city place with Mommy and Daddy."

"You don't have to believe me, but I'm just trying to get home."

"Shut up, punk. How much cash do you have on you?"

"Please," I said. "My train card has twenty bucks left on it, and I have thirty dollars in my pocket. You can have it."

"You're forgetting something. That's a fine gold necklace you're wearing, but it would look a lot better on me. Hand it over!"

My fear was suddenly replaced with sadness. It wasn't *any* gold necklace. It was one of the most special things I owned. It had been bought for me by one of the most special people in my life, my Aunt Donna.

Donna was no ordinary person—the only one in my family that I trusted and respected. Despite her humble beginnings, she had worked a few jobs and saved her money. She would take me places and let me spend time at her home. She was more like a mother than my own. I felt a stabbing pain in my chest, as if someone was squeezing my heart. The money meant nothing to me, those thugs could gladly take it, but the necklace was a valuable piece of my past. There was no way I could replace it. "Listen—you can have everything, but please leave me with this necklace. It means a lot to me. It was a present from my aunt."

"Oh, you're breaking my heart," the tall thug drawled, mocking me. "Your aunt, huh? Well, tell auntie to get you another one."

He lunged at me, and I looked behind me and saw Ralphie kneeling down. Things began to blur. The last thing I recall was the feeling of kicking feet and punching fists before I slipped into a velvet darkness.

When I regained consciousness, a terrible stench greeted my nostrils. I looked up and recognized the man who had been talking to himself when I first entered the station. However, now he was talking to me. "Hey buddy, you OK? You look like hell."

I felt like saying, "I look like you smell," but I was trying to be nice to this Good Samaritan. "I'll be all right."

"I saw 'em running down the platform. This place is a sewer." He stared at me. "Your lip is bleeding."

I tried blotting it with my left hand.

He reached into his pocket and pulled out a filthy handkerchief. "Here, use this."

"No, thanks." My head was splitting.

"Then fuck you." He began walking away, mumbling to himself. "Ungrateful kids. They ain't got any manners. Little bastards."

A moment later, he turned around and yelled, "Got a dollar for me?"

"Sorry," I replied. "They took everything I had."

He continued on his walk, commiserating with his imaginary companion.

Forcing myself to stand up was the easy part. The hard part was bringing my hand to my neck to feel whether the gold chain was still there. It was gone and, with it, a piece of my heart.

Fortunately, I had hidden a twenty-dollar bill in my inner pocket. I reached inside and found that the pocket was empty. "Bastards took everything."

I struggled back to the original platform just in time to see a man in a transit uniform.

"What happened to you, mister?" He looked at me suspiciously.

I was not looking to get the police involved, and I certainly not to spend time in any more hospitals. I had seen enough nurses to last me the rest of my life. "All I need to do is get home, sir. When is the next train to the city?"

"I'm opening up the fare booth now. Follow me. The

train should be coming within fifteen minutes."

"What time is it?" I asked.

"It's 4:00 a.m. Rush hour will be starting soon."

It was difficult to believe that I had spent so many hours suffering in a place called Jubilee Junction. I limped along behind him, my shirt pulled up over my lip.

At the fare booth, he handed me a roll of paper towels. "Here you go. Clean yourself up—you'll scare the passengers, know what I mean? . . . You're not in any trouble, are you?"

"No, I'll be all right. I really appreciate your help, sir."

"You seem like a nice kid. There's a lot of riff-raff that hangs out in this station at night. You got to be really careful."

"Don't worry." I almost laughed—the warning was a little bit late.

"The train will be here shortly. Take care of yourself, OK?"

I stumbled over to the bench and began to take deep breaths. The ordeal was over. Once more I reached up to my neck, hoping that, magically, the necklace would be back in place. The sound of the approaching train propelled me to my feet.

Once inside, I looked around at this morning group of passengers. Most were dressed in suits. They probably

had fancy office jobs, I surmised. I felt painfully conspicuous. I could feel eyes sneaking glances at the bloody,
bruised, handicapped kid in their midst. I felt like yelling
out to them. I felt like telling them my whole miserable
story. I wanted to let them know about my rotten childhood, my accident, my uphill battle to recovery, and the
beating I had just taken. I wanted to scream at them,
"Could *you* have survived what I have survived?"

Instead, I closed my eyes until the conductor an-
nounced my stop.

CHAPTER 20

MY MODEST APARTMENT LOOKED palatial when I got to it, and my bed was calling me. It was time to give my bruised mind and body a nice long rest. The next day was Saturday, and after turning my cell phone off, my plans were merely to sleep.

I lay down on my bed and began trying to find a comfortable position, but there was none. My body ached. It was agony. All I wanted to do was drift off into that wonderful netherworld and forget the excruciating ordeal. Yet this was an excruciating ordeal of a different kind.

"There must be some pain medication around," I mumbled. I was growing frantic. Ah, yes, the pills that I'd been given at Fastline! Flinging open my drawer, I spotted the small orange vial. The directions read *Take two as needed.*

I popped three. The noise in the streets began to fade as I lay in bed, staring at the old picture of my family that was mounted on the wall near my bed. The Anthony smiling at me appeared to be about five years old. He had two hands.

Strangely, as I stared at the picture, I became aware of the wall moving towards me. What was happening?

"Hey, Tony," a young boy's voice called out, startling me. "How long are you going to hog that swing? Give someone else a chance!"

"Shut up. I just got on this thing."

"You got on this thing a long time ago. We're supposed to take turns."

"Oh, yeah?" I snapped. "And where's that written?"

"Right here." I felt myself being pushed off the swing. I was falling and falling but not hitting ground. It was as if I were going into an abyss.

"Help!" I screamed, looking up at the disappearing swing in the distance. There was a man standing there looking down at me. It was my father.

"Tony, get up here. Are you going to let that little bastard push you around? Get up here and start acting like a man."

"I'm coming, Dad!" I tried to climb up out of the hole,

but the earth kept slipping through my fingers. "I can't—"

My father screamed, "I said get *over* here!"

The hole disappeared, and I was standing in front of my old man. His glance was stern.

He turned to the other boy who was swinging happily. "Get off that swing, you little punk."

The swing stopped abruptly.

"Don't you know that you never hit a guy from behind? Get over here and fight like a real man." My father grabbed us both. We stood there staring nervously at one another.

"Now, let's see who's the real man!"

I lifted my right hand with determination. But as my arm flew through the air, it got slower and slower. It was as if my hand would never reach my adversary. I looked at my arm in bewilderment. It was gone. I felt weak and sick to my stomach.

My opponent took advantage of my hesitation, and I fell to the ground. I closed my eyes, afraid to see the expression on my father's face.

When I opened them, I was no longer in the playground but lying on the floor at Jubilee Junction, and the thugs who had kicked my ass were running away.

"Good job, Ralphie. You are now a member of the Night Hawks."

I rolled over and realized, to my horror, that I was on the subway tracks, watching the headlights of a train in the distance. It was coming towards me. I felt paralyzed. I began screaming, but it seemed as if my voice was gone. I covered my eyes and waited as death hurtled toward me.

When I finally mustered the courage to open my eyes, I was surprised to find myself on the floor of my apartment. Perspiration had formed a pool around my body, which was shaking in pain.

The clock was ticking as if someone had turned up the volume. I glanced over to see that it was 10:00 a.m. Laughter drifted upwards from the street.

"*Damn* it. I'll *never* get the sleep I need. There must be some sleeping pills somewhere around this place."

I flung my drawer open. The gods were taking pity on me: A bottle of Nyquil caught my eye. After a generous gulp, I draped a towel over the window and a pillow over my face, and drifted off into a peaceful slumber.

When my eyes opened again, the clock caught my attention. Ten o'clock! Was my mind going? But I looked again and noticed the small *p.m.* next to the numbers. My sleep had lasted twelve hours.

The aches were still there, and my head felt groggy. I splashed some cold water on my face, determined not to sleep any more of my life away. Thank God it was still

Saturday, and tomorrow would be another day to recuperate.

The weekend quickly slipped into Monday, and another hectic day greeted me. I'd mastered the routine. It was as if someone had wound me up, and I went automatically from school to physical therapy and then to work. My grades were good, and the job was easy, but boredom had begun to blanket me. Catering Needs was a dead-end situation, and the money sucked.

"Maybe I should get a job on an assembly line for some stimulation," I grumbled as I went through my robotic routine. Money became my focus. I wanted a well-paying, satisfying career, not a monotonous, mediocre job.

To add to the frustration, I seemed to be hitting a wall with Dr. Wegman's office. For two months I'd been calling, and for two months I'd gotten the same response: "Sorry, Tony, we're working on it. We still haven't gotten the final authorization."

"What do you mean?" My impatience was reaching a crescendo. "Working on what? I thought everything was settled."

"The cast is made, but we just have to be certain that we will be reimbursed." The receptionist tried to calm me down. "Don't worry, Tony, it shouldn't be much longer."

Patience was not one of my virtues. "Please see if you can move this thing along? You don't know what it feels like to be without an arm."

"We're doing our best. It's easy to get stuck in the world of red tape."

I wondered whether the receptionist was trying to be funny, but I was not laughing. "I'm sure you know what you're doing." My sarcasm was apparent.

THE END OF MY THIRD SEMESTER WAS QUICKLY approaching. School would be out for the summer, and I planned to enroll in summer school in an effort to lighten my fall course load. I also planned to do a thorough job search.

While I was sitting in my Monday morning class, my cell phone rang, waking up a sleeping student in the back of the room. It was Dr. Wegman's office smiling at me from the caller I.D. Excusing myself, I ran into the hall.

The receptionist's voice was like music. "I've got good news for you, Anthony—we've received the final authorization and are prepared to move forward."

Thoughts of Jubilee Junction tarnished my good mood. "Could we make the appointment a little earlier than last time?"

"No problem, Tony. Come in at 3:00. It shouldn't

take very long."

The trip to Dr. Wegman's office went off without a hitch. I had no encounters en route and, for the first time, the doctor's waiting room was nearly empty.

The receptionist smiled. "This is a light day for the doctor. He'll be with you shortly. Follow me."

I sat anxiously awaiting Dr. Wegman's entrance. Was this the day that my new hand would find its new home? How long I'd awaited this moment.

He entered wearing a big smile that I recognized as the smile of reimbursement. "Sorry that this has taken so long, Tony. It's hard to navigate these bureaucracies, but I've become an expert."

"As long as things have worked out." Nothing was going to upset me—or so I thought. However, as I watched the doctor, my eyes landed on an eerie device that he was removing from a plastic bag.

"What on earth is that?" I stared at the contraption.

"It's a check socket. Don't get upset. This is a long way from the final product. The reason it's clear is so we can tell if there are any issues with the fit, or imperfections in the prosthesis.

The whole thing looked like an imperfection.

"Tony, the finished product will not look like this. But we can't rush the procedure," he said to reassure me.

I stared at the device. It was a clear mold that resembled a hand, but you could see all the inner workings. The battery was visible, and so were the wires. I was breathing deeply in an effort to ward off my anxiety.

"Make sure you take this to therapy with you, and work with it there," Dr. Wegman continued in his chipper demeanor. "Tony, you will come to appreciate this. Remember my words."

We scheduled another appointment, and I left with a heavy heart and a hideous hand in a plastic bag. Maybe I'd wear it in the apartment, but certainly not in public. Nobody was going to see this thing. Since the accident, I'd had enough stares aimed in my direction. I'd had enough jokes made at my expense. This supposed "hand" was a magnet for ridicule, and I was not going to invite any.

CHAPTER 21

WEEKENDS OFFERED ME NO RESPITE, since I had stopped going out. In fact, doing so no longer even tempted me. My aim was to excel in school and find myself a well-paying job, and this was not going to be accomplished falling off a bar stool drunk.

One typical Friday evening in the Risoli apartment, my nose was buried in a textbook when the sound of the buzzer startled me. "Who is it?" I asked.

"Kyle and Robbie. Do you remember us?"

"What the hell are you guys doing here?" My voice might have sounded angry, but underneath the surprise, I was happy to hear from them.

"T., you going to let us up?"

"Sure. Hang on."

The sound of footsteps on the stairs was strangely comforting, too.

"What's been happening?" Kyle asked. "Why don't you ever answer your phone? You've become a total recluse."

Robbie added, "You know what they say about all work and no play, T. You don't want to become a dull boy, do you?"

"We are the rescue party," Kyle declares. "Your worries are over."

"It's really great to see you guys. Maybe I *have* been overdoing it. Between work, school, and therapy, it seems as if there's no time for anything else. I was afraid that, if I started partying, I'd lose my focus."

"Well, tonight you're taking a break."

Kyle's eye caught my check socket. "What the hell is that?" He looked horrified. "Tony, are you going to be appearing in a horror flick?"

"No jokes, please. I'm going through enough with this thing."

Rob looked apologetic. "That's not your new arm, is it?"

"No. This is only the first stage. I have to get used to it before they can make the finished product."

"How does it work?"

I demonstrated the hand while my friends sat there transfixed.

Rob interrupted the performance. "Let's go out for a drink."

The thought was extremely appealing. As we ambled down the flights, Kyle said sheepishly, "I can't wait to see it when it's done. Sorry about the comments. They were stupid. I have one question, however—will the battery be showing when it is finished?"

That was a good question. "I'll have to ask my doctor."

My friends were right. The break was just what I needed. I'd almost forgotten how to have a good time. They say that there are some things you never forget, like riding a bike. Drinking definitely belongs on that list. Before long, I was laughing so hard I almost fell off my bar stool. It seemed as if the party had just begun when the bartender yelled, "Last call."

"You don't know how great it was to see you guys tonight," I told them when they were leaving; I was choked up with emotion.

"Then do us a favor, Tony—pick up your fucking phone from now on."

"No problem."

I guess I'd been so distracted that I'd forgotten how important my friends were to me. I slept soundly that night.

The days that followed had an added element, my check socket. I knew that Dr. Wegman wanted me to get used to it, but my resistance was too powerful.

The hand went with me to physical therapy where I learned what it could and couldn't do. Then the hand went back to the apartment, where I'd wear it in private. But whenever I went out, it remained at home.

DURING MY NEXT APPOINTMENT, Kyle's question popped into my head. "Dr. Wegman, will the battery be visible on the final product?"

"Don't worry, it will all be hidden once it's finished."

"And when will that be?" I dreaded the answer.

"It should be ready in a month."

My mouth dropped.

"Tony, I know it feels as if it's taking a very long time, but you're coming down the home stretch. Cheer up."

He was right. There in the distance, though still a blur, waited my new hand and my new life. I put a smile on my face and left the office.

In the weeks that followed, I eased up on my routine a bit and saw my friends on weekends. It made the weeks a lot more bearable, and time, in its mysterious way, stopped dragging. In fact, when the call came from Dr. Wegman's office, I was surprised that a whole month had gone by.

"It's here!" The receptionist sounded as happy telling me the news as I felt hearing it. "Are you available the day after tomorrow?"

I cannot say that Jubilee Junction resembled a home away from home, but a lot of my anxiety had dissipated. I had by then long committed the train schedule, and when the corridors and toll booths were closed. Yet I knew that a bit of prudent caution was necessary, so I requested an early appointment.

The following day, I got a surprise call from Dr. Wegman's office. "I made a mistake," the receptionist said. She sounded apologetic. "I scheduled you for the day when Dr. Wegman goes to Beldale Hospital. Why don't you just meet him there? Then you and the physical therapist can be present to greet the arm."

This was indeed great news, and it called for a celebration. That night, I treated myself to a falafel from the downstairs sandwich shop. A man in a wheelchair passed me en route, and we smiled at one another. I wondered what kind of turmoil *he* had experienced. Maybe someday I'll be in a position to help people like that man, I thought.

The next day, my thoughts were completely scattered. I was trying to get everything accomplished and be at Beldale Hospital on time to meet Dr. Wegman. When I got to the subway, I realized that, in my haste, I had forgotten my subway card. Because funds were running low, I put my body in reverse and headed back to the apartment.

But as I approached my block, I ran into a big commotion. The street had been blocked off, and there were cops on the scene.

One stopped me. "Sorry, police activity. I cannot let you through here."

"But I live here," I said.

"If you wait here, I'll get the sergeant to speak to you."

"But I'm going to be late for my appointment at Beldale Hospital. I don't need to talk to any sergeant."

There was something uncomfortably familiar about what was happening. Had I been in this situation before? Ah, yes, I thought, making sense of the haze, my mind traveling back in time to an incident that had occurred when I was about eleven years old.

After a tedious day at school, I'd returned to my home, only to be greeted by a frowning father. My mother had been standing a few inches behind him.

"Sit down, Tony, we have to talk to you."

"But I haven't done anything," I said. The cat jumped

on the table, and my father swatted him to the floor. "Listen, Anthony, don't lie to me. Where are the bikes?"

"Bikes? What are you talking about?"

"You know damn well what I'm talking about. But before I hear any more of your BS, there is one thing you had better get straight, and get it straight right now. You must never lie to your parents. I am on your side, just remember that."

I looked down at the floor.

"I heard from two detectives earlier. You and your friend Zack were reported by some locals for stealing bikes from a house in town. The detectives said that, because of the situation, they're going to be coming to the house to talk with you."

I started sweating guilty drops of perspiration. It was too late for lying. My father's words "I am on your side" kept playing in my mind.

"Tony, please don't forget that I am your father. I will always be there for you, no matter what you do. The only thing I insist on is that you never lie to me."

"We did it, Dad," I confessed through the lump in my throat. "But I swear it was Zack's idea. He took the bikes and was going to sell them."

My father grew quiet as his expression softened. "I believe you, son."

I will never forget that feeling. Suddenly I felt incredibly loved. I felt protected and I felt grateful as I choked back the tears.

"I never liked that Zack," my mother chimed in. "He's a thirteen-year-old punk who's always trying to act like a big shot. You see, Joe? I *told* you that I didn't want Tony hanging out with him."

"Maria, now is not the time for this. Just let me be alone with Tony."

My mother left the room.

"Thanks for being honest with me, son—I don't care about the bikes at this point. When these detectives get here, don't say anything. I've got your back."

"Kid!" A loud voice had brought me back to the present. "I have some questions for you." The man standing in front of me was Sergeant O'Shea, although, as he rambled on, I'd still been able to hear my father's voice telling me my rights. *Don't answer any questions.*

The advice had been well taken. It was bad enough that this nonsense was making me late for my appointment.

"Look at my arm," I said, and waved it in front of him. "My doctor is waiting to fit a prosthetic, and I don't have any time for questions."

I headed upstairs, got the damn transit card, and left

the building. One foot followed the other heading to the subway. Nobody called after me, and nobody followed. Perhaps they had taken pity on the one-armed young man. Perhaps they too knew my rights.

Subway card clutched tightly, I completed my trip to Beldale Hospital and shoed up only fifteen minutes late for my appointment.

"Tony, I was worried about you." Dr. Wegman's voice was warm and kind. "Is everything O.K?"

"Sure, no problem. There was some police activity on my block that slowed me up. I hope I haven't thrown off your schedule."

"Not at all. Are you ready for the big unveiling?" He was holding a black cloth bag. "It came out great, Tony." He proceeded to unleash the prosthetic device from its container. "Here she is!"

Yes, there she was, the device that was supposed to be the answer to all my problems and make me whole again.

The word "nervous" does not come close to what I was feeling. It was difficult to even focus my eyes on the hand, my expectations were soaring. Dr. Wegman passed it to me.

"Whoa, this is heavy, heavier than the socket."

Before he could respond, I turned the device and noticed that the battery was protruding from the forearm.

"But, Doc, I thought you said that they'd be able to hide this battery." My voice cracked. From the corner of my eye, I saw Rosalie's face drop.

Dr. Wegman began stammering, "Uh, uh. . .let me call them. In the meantime, put it on and see if it works properly."

As I struggled with the unfamiliar appendage, he picked up the clinic phone and began dialing the manufacturer. When he was transferred to the correct department, he put the call on speaker phone.

"What was the patient's name?"

"Rissoli. Transradial amputee on the right side."

"Hold on." Elevator music filled in the silence. While the music meandered irritatingly, I'd begun experimenting with the device. As promised, the hand opened and closed. To my surprise, I discovered that controlling it was easy.

Rosalie placed a cone-shaped object in front of me and told me to pick it up.

I reached down. "Wow, I can do it!" She and I were both beaming with accomplishment. She was feeling good about her part in my success, and I was feeling grateful that the arm had some merit.

The elevator music came to a jarring halt and a voice blared from the speaker phone. "Alan, are you still there?"

"Of course," Dr. Wegman responded.

"Just checked with the fabrication department, and according to our lead technician, this was the best set-up they could provide. Unfortunately, it was due to the length of the patient's limb."

Dr. Wegman was visibly annoyed. "I've had patients with similar residual limbs, and you've always been able to hide the battery."

He turned off the speaker; I wasn't privy to the rest of conversation.

Rosalie turned to me with words of reassurance. And though I feigned understanding, I really did not understand this turn of events.

Dr. Wegman hung up the phone. "You'll get used to it, Tony. Take it home and practice with it. Wear it as much as you can. I'll call you if something can be done to remedy the glitch."

He laid a piece of paper in front of me. "Oh, yes, and before you leave, please sign on the dotted line. It's for insurance purposes. We've got to get paid." He looked embarrassed.

I left the hospital with my new arm and headed for the train. My mind still had not adjusted to its appearance, and entering the subway car did nothing to bolster my morale. Were people staring at me? Was it in my mind?

"Mister, what's the matter with your hand?"

"Shh," a blushing mother whispered, trying to quiet her youngster.

It was too late. The comment had brought more glances in my direction, and I felt more conspicuous than before. Though my body was feeling physically comfortable, my mind was a psychological wreck.

Prior to the arrival of the prosthetic, I'd been able to hide my limb under my sleeve, but now it was out in public for all to see. Was it growing larger? Was I totally losing my mind?

I walked back to my place with my head down. Arriving at my door, I encountered a new challenge. Could my new hand open the door? The key fell to the floor. The limited dexterity guaranteed failure. After a few more tries, my left hand came to the rescue, and my heart sank.

So, within thirty minutes of getting the prosthetic device, my world was falling apart. It was as if all hope had been crushed. There was only one option left for me. I put the device back in the black bag and shoved it under my bed.

CHAPTER 22

A LTHOUGH I WAS FRUSTRATED and disappointed with the prosthetic device, there were other loose ends in my life that needed some attention, too. One of them was my job at Catering Needs. Day after day I would do phone work. It was beyond boring.

"Catering Needs—can I help you?"

"Catering Needs—we cater to your needs."

"Catering Needs—I am about to strangle myself."

A well-trained monkey could have done what I was doing. Was it was because of my disability that my duties were so limited? In the suburbs, I had been given a great deal of responsibility, but, then again, those had been the days when Anthony Risoli had two hands. What genius ever said two heads are better than one? If he'd said "hands," it would have made more sense.

I sat at the reception desk daydreaming. My boss's voice startled me.

"Tony, don't you hear me?"

"Oh, sorry, Mr. Harris— have a lot on my mind."

"Weren't you supposed to get your new arm? It would help with your work here. In fact, I could probably give you some more challenging assignments."

What did he mean by challenging? Did he feel that I was incapable of performing the simplest of tasks because I had only one hand? I wanted to quit his stupid job but, instead, I politely replied, "No, sir, it's not ready yet. There are still some issues that have to be worked out."

It was difficult to keep up the cheerful facade when everything in my life was pulling me down, screaming failure. Maybe I *was* a failure. Maybe I was kidding myself with my grandiose plans and ideas. Nothing was working out.

It was time to leave this dreadful place and go home to my sanctuary. As I passed the corner bar, it seemed to be pulling me inside. Ah, the perfect medicine. A drink or two might numb the pain.

I was greeted by an attractive blonde bartender who took my order. As I stared at her face, the image of my ex-girlfriend, Jenn, superimposed itself. It was difficult for me to admit how much I missed her. We had had so many good times. I longed for her, and the pain in my gut grew more intense. Loneliness and misery sat down with me on that bar stool. My mind wandered back to the days before my accident. Why hadn't I appreciated what I had? How deeply I missed my family and my friends. I had neglected them all. When I did drop home, I was always distracted, always looking for a reason to leave early.

"Sorry, Mom, but I have a paper due at school." The looks of disappointment haunted me.

What had I done? I'd made a mess of my life, that's what.

"You are a failure, Risoli," I said out loud.

"Excuse me?" The bartender looked in my direction. "Are you talking to me?"

"No, I'm sorry," I responded. "I was just thinking out loud."

She smiled and continued pouring the drinks, and I continued sitting as if I were glued to the bar stool. There was nowhere to go and nobody to go there with. Most of all, I dreaded going up the stairs to my apartment alone.

"You remind me of my son," an attractive older woman said, beginning a friendly dialogue with me. "I haven't seen him in years and I miss him." Her slurred words were strangely comforting. I was grateful that someone was talking to me. I wondered how much she had been drinking. She rambled on and on. I cannot for the life of me recall what we talked about, but the longer we did, the better she looked. During the entire conversation, I kept my right arm hidden under my shirt. I wanted so desperately to appear normal.

The lights went on. It was closing time, and as I got up to leave, the woman kissed my cheek and extended her right arm. I drunkenly extended my stump. She did not turn away but, instead, seemed intrigued. "Where are you going now?" she asked.

"Home. Do you want to come?" The liquor had made us fast friends, and as she climbed the staircase with me, her head flopped onto my shoulder.

"You sure are cute." Her arm went around my waist.

The last thing I remember was putting a movie in the DVD player and lying down.

WAKING UP THE NEXT DAY WAS NOT EASY. My head ached, and my vision was fuzzy. I looked around my room. My new companion was gone, but that wasn't all. The room was a wreck. My movies were gone! All my dresser drawers were open, and some of my belongings were strewn on the floor. Though my head was splitting, I could still put two and two together. I had been robbed!

That bitch had *robbed me!* My heart began to hurt as much as my head. The pit of emptiness inside was now bottomless. I wished I had died that day on the State Thruway.

I will never know what came over me at that point, but suddenly I felt a sense of panic about my new arm. Had that been stolen too? Even though I'd hated it, cold fear gripped me.

"Please, God, let it be there."

I can hardly describe the sense of relief I felt when I saw the device nestled safely in its black container.

You're a lunatic, Risoli! Why do you care about that hideous thing?

"Who said that?" I began searching around my room. Had I lost more than my possessions? Had I lost my mind?

"My cash stash!" I began shaking. Had she found the money I'd hidden behind the pipe?

I crawled under the sink. The money was there. I took a deep breath and staggered over to the bathroom mirror. "Snap out of this!" I snarled at the red-eyed reflection. "Get a grip."

My heart was pounding. These emotional ups and downs were driving me insane. And equally as bad, or maybe worse, they were causing me to be vulnerable to predators.

Perhaps a cold shower would ease my troubled mind. As the water cascaded down my aching body, it was joined by tears flowing freely from my eyes. I no longer cared whether I was acting like a man or not. I no longer cared if my father would have approved. All I knew is that my heart was breaking, my life was crumbling, and I needed to release the pain and frustration that were exploding inside me. It felt so good to release all those pent-up emotions. And when the tears subsided, it was as if I had cleansed both my body and my soul.

As I stood in the shower, feeling freer than I'd felt in months, my mind began taking a selective inventory. First I'd been mugged on the subway, and now I'd been robbed in my own apartment. Perhaps Mr. Harris was not the only one whose behavior had been shaped by my missing arm. Perhaps I was being targeted as a victim. I thought of Edmund and the other amputees I'd met. Had they had similar experiences? And, if they had, where had *they* turned? Had anyone been available to help them?

I thought about the Disability Department at school. Supposedly they had had a club about five years before that advocated for the rights of the disabled. Why was it no longer in existence? What had happened to it, and could it be brought back to life? It was at this moment that a realization thwacked me on the head. I, Anthony Risoli, was going to revive the club. I would start immediately after the weekend.

CHAPTER 23

ONDAY COULD NOT HAVE ARRIVED soon enough. My excitement was palpable. My life now had a mission, and it was clear.

I got to the school an hour early and waited outside the office of the Director of Disability Services.

"Tony, what are you doing here so early?" Mrs. Wright was rushing to her office. "You cannot believe how much work I've got waiting for me! I never expected to see anyone here. Is everything OK?"

My ideas poured from my mouth as Beth Wright sat in rapt attention.

"Tony," she at last said, "this sounds *great!* I would *love* to start the club again. I even know other faculty members who would be eager to assist you in chartering it. Please understand that my time is stretched to the limit these days, but this is definitely a priority. Speak to my secretary and set up an appointment. In the meantime, go to the Student Government Department and see what information they can give you. They have a whole protocol that must be followed for setting up this club. There will be a lot of forms to fill out."

"Thanks, Mrs. Wright." I started to leave.

"Tony, you've started my day off with a smile."

"Mine, too."

In fact, my whole being was smiling. I sprinted down the hall to Math, a class I normally despised. Yet that day, something had shifted. My attitude was different, and suddenly the class seemed enjoyable.

After Math, it was off to English Journalism. Professor Rally noticed the change in me. "You seem unusually cheerful today, Tony."

"I feel great. I'm headed in a new direction."

"Going to the West Coast?" His sense of humor took some getting used to.

"Nope, something better than that. I want to start a student club that promotes the interests of students with disabilities."

"Tony, that's a *fantastic* idea. I don't know if you believe in coincidences, but this is an incredible case of synchronicity. I used to be the editor of a magazine that focused on disability issues. We wound up getting shut down because the funds dried up. Perhaps it's time to find the money. See me after class, Tony."

All through the professor's lecture, my mind raced. Ideas were turning around in my head. A new club was being birthed, and I was preparing for its arrival.

When class ended and I again approached him, we spoke as he gathered his lecture materials. "Tony, I know all about the protocol for your student club. First of all, you'll need a faculty sponsor. Also you will have to have five chartered members even before submitting the paperwork. Do you have anyone in mind to sponsor your club?"

I mustered up my courage. "Would you be willing to do it?"

"I thought you'd never ask," he chuckled. "I'd love to help you as much as I can. Meet me after class on Thursday, and we'll go over the paperwork from Student Government."

"Great. I'm heading over there right now."

The packet was larger than I'd thought it'd be, and I sat down on a bench and began to peruse the contents. There, in bold letters, was a paragraph explaining the five-member requirement to make it an official club.

How would I go about securing five people? Perhaps I could make fliers and distribute them.

The following day, I headed to the Disability Department for my appointment with Mrs. Wright. In my enthusiasm, I arrived twenty-five minutes early. I could not contain myself and began sharing my idea with the secretary. Not surprisingly, she loved the idea.

"I remember the club we used to have. It must have been over three years ago. The students seemed to get a lot from it. I know people were very upset when it was disbanded."

"I need five active members to start it. I was thinking of making some fliers and distributing them to the students."

"You can use the printer in this office," she volunteered. "But better yet, why don't we make a sign-up sheet, and I'll display it in a prominent place. This way, all the students will see it when they file through this office. It can get very busy here."

The phone rang. "Mrs. Wright will see you now."

After our meeting, I rushed off to class, but my mind was no longer on my studies. The club had taken up residence in my head.

Before leaving the building, I went over to the Disability Office. How could I go home without checking the status of the sign-up sheet?

I bet it's empty, I thought.

However, when I got to the office, I noticed that the secretary was wearing a wide grin. She pointed to the sheet. There were already three names on it, and it was only the first day.

"Oh! I almost forgot about myself," I said, and added my name to the list.

"I only need one more name."

"You'll get more than that, Tony. You're off to an impressive start."

The following day, two more names joined the four assembled ones, and by the end of the week, I'd met with each perspective member. We were ready to finalize the paperwork. We called a meeting for that Tuesday and, after much deliberation, decided to coin our club The Difference Makers.

One day at our weekly meeting, I saw Dr. Wegman's name light up my cell phone. "How are you doing Tony? I hope you're feeling comfortable with the arm by now."

Oh, no! I thought. I had nearly forgotten the poor arm, hidden under my bed. My new club had been occupying most of my thoughts. "Great," I lied.

"Good to hear that. Listen, Tony, I'm doing a lecture at the City University. I'll be addressing group of hand surgeons on upper-extremity prosthetics. I'd love to have you showcase the hand and explain how it works. If you accept, there'll be a $100.00 check for your time."

My mind traveled back to the last time such an offer had been made to me. It seemed like a lifetime ago, when the delectable Marly told me about an opportunity that, coincidentally, paid the same fee. That had worked out well, and I'd been able to network with the occupational therapists. Even though this appeared more demanding, I accepted the challenge.

"I'd be happy to do it."

"It's in two weeks, Tony, at Beldale." I brushed aside any self-doubt. If I was going to realize my dreams, I'd better stop wrestling with life.

I might add that, at the end of two weeks, I'd added another success to my expanding list.

THE DIFFERENCE MAKERS IS LIVING UP to its name.

We attracted both students and faculty members who were eager to modernize the college's awareness of people with disabilities. Word spread, and before long, we were working closely with other colleges and universities in the area.

I think I speak for all the members when I say that the meetings were our favorite parts of the week. The only problem was that they never felt long enough. Our enrollment soon spread, and the members were always bursting with anecdotes and ideas.

Branching out was our next step. We began to sponsor events in which tutorials were held demonstrating the strides that had been made in assistive devices for the disabled. One such miraculous device was a computer that read to the blind, interpreting whatever text was placed before him or her. It introduced a whole universe into the lives of people who had lost their vision.

The club was the talk of the campus and, I am sure, other campuses in the area. As the enrollment grew, and the list of sponsors along with it, my mind was once again racing.

"Why not turn this concept into a *non-profit organization?*" I asked one day.

There was obviously a huge need for this kind of service. I recalled the day long, long ago when I sat in Dr. Wegman's office, perusing the magazines. "Yes," I said quietly to myself, "that was the day the idea first passed through my mind." But now, the dream was close to becoming a reality. All my dreams had been realized when I had applied myself. Why should this be any different? *Ampunation:* The word flashed across the screen of my mind.

I approached Professor Rally. Once again, he was the ideal man with whom to confer. "Tony," he said, "this is perfect. I can supply you with a host of people I know will be willing to donate to your corporation."

CHAPTER 24

THEY CALL GRADUATION "COMMENCEMENT," and for me it was truly a new beginning. Though I had to painfully say goodbye to Hoover College, I joyously bid Catering Needs a fond *adieu*. It was time to toss off the security blanket of school and enter what is somewhat euphemistically called the Real World.

I had over a hundred members in my club by then, and donations of twenty thousand dollars for assistive technology through sponsorships and the help of student contributors.

My schedule had become nearly unmanageable, and the phone never stopped ringing. As I stood in front of the bathroom mirror, I recalled the time a bleary-eyed drunk had squinted back at me, yelling, "Failure." I was seeing a bright-eyed young man in that mirror.

"Are you ready for me, world?"

EPILOGUE

S THIS THE END OF ANTHONY RISOLI'S STORY? *No, not at all. He now sits behind a large, impressive desk. The company that he formed, Ampunation, has acquired a life of its own, and it had grown and grown, realizing its promise. A staff has been hired to keep up with the activity.*

Testimonials inundate his mailbox. They are tributes to him from peoples whose lives have been changed. They are praises for him from people who were ready to put an end to their agony.

I am hoping that Anthony's story will serve as an inspiration to you and to everyone who reads it.

I waved good-bye to Anthony and stopped one moment to read a message on the wall from Elbert Hubbard:

"Down in their hearts, wise people know the truth, the only way to help yourself is to help others."

www.ingramcontent.com/pod-product-compliance
Lightning Source LLC
Chambersburg PA
CBHW021104090426
42738CB00006B/499